THE MENTAL HOSPITAL AND HUMAN SERVICES

THE MENTAL HOSPITAL AND HUMAN SERVICES

Herbert C. Schulberg, Ph.D.
United Community Planning Corporation and Harvard Medical School

and

Frank Baker, Ph.D.
Harvard Medical School

Behavioral Publications
New York

Library of Congress Catalog Number 74-668
ISBN: 0-87705-138-0

BEHAVIORAL PUBLICATIONS, Inc.
72 Fifth Avenue
New York, New York 10011

Printed in the United States of America

Library of Congress Cataloging in Publication Data

Schulberg, Herbert C
The mental hospital and human services.

Bibliography: p.
1. Psychiatric hospitals. 2. Community mental health services. I. Baker, Frank, 1936- joint author. II. Title. [DNLM: 1. Community mental health services. 2. Hospitals, Psychiatric. WM30 S385m 1974]
RC439.S387 362.2'1 74-668

For the patients and staff of
Boston State Hospital,
and all others who struggle to make
the inhumane more humane

Contents

PREFACE

The nature and quality of mental health programs have undergone major transitions during the past decade. Even from the perspective of those advocating more revolutionary and far-reaching changes, there can be little doubt that treatment of the mentally ill in 1974 differs considerably from the caregiving patterns of 10 years ago. The concept of comprehensive services provided within local catchment areas has won widespread acceptance, the ideology of integrated human services is developing a prominence akin to that of community mental health beliefs in the late 1960's, new caregiving arrangements are offering clients services beyond those psychiatric ones available in community mental health centers, and the large mental hospital's traditionally central role has been altered or diminished.

All changes, even those that are progressive, create systemic reverberations, however, and profound problems still exist in serving the mentally ill. The increased utilization of community-based resources has focused public attention upon service gaps which long went unnoticed, contemporary fiscal bases and manpower patterns which must be developed, and complex and politically sensitive decisions which must be made about the mental hospital's future if the full array of human services is to be available for clients in distress. In brief, the past decade's changes have been awesome in their aspirations but still unfulfilled in their outcomes. What are the reasons for this state of affairs, and what conceptual frameworks can best help to render intelligent national and local program transitions?

As participants in and observers of the changing mental health scene, we have written this book to convey our understanding of the preceding questions. Since our personal roles during the past years have included major planning and research responsibilities, our perspective clearly is action-oriented as well as analytic. The first author (HCS) served from 1963 to 1965 as a staff member of the Massachusetts Mental Health Planning Project, from 1965 to 1969 as Head of a Laboratory of Community Psychiatry, Harvard Medical School research program studying Boston State Hospital's evolution from mental hospital to community mental health functions, and most recently as Director of the Massachusetts Mental Hospital Planning Project. The second author (FB) has been engaged in consultation, as well as teaching and research in the field of community mental health since he joined the faculty of the Harvard Medical School Laboratory of Community Psychiatry in 1965. As Head of the Program Research Unit and Director of the Organizational Systems Research and Evaluation Section of the Laboratory of Community Psychiatry, he continues to focus on helping through consultation to plan, manage, and evaluate changes in ongoing human service systems, as well as studying changing organizational systems operating under different conditions.

Given our longstanding interests and activities in this field, how could we succinctly portray within the covers of a single book the historic ebb and flow of societal and professional concerns for the mentally ill? How in this volume could we analyze for their unique as well as collective impact upon patient care such interrelated strands as legislative mandates and sanctions, organizational needs and maintenance concerns, expanded client expectations, shifting professional roles, and evolving clinical ideologies and technologies? The candid answer is that we could not fully capture all relevant descriptive and analytic perspectives within one treatise, particularly since our goal was that of simultaneously examining the dynamics and consequences of program change in breadth as well as in depth. As a result, the following book is recognizedly less comprehensive than we had initially envisioned it would be. Nevertheless, recent developments on the mental health scene are of such historic significance that even partial efforts to capture their subtleties and complexities seem warranted as a contribution to the mental health practitioner's and social scientist's grasp of program and organizational change.

It is, thus, within a framework of seeking simultaneously to portray program changes at their broadest as well as at their most detailed levels that our book traces the key events and factors which in the past decade have shifted the mental health caregiving system's emphasis from institutional, inpatient services to community-based, outpatient ones. Section I presents the generic issues faced by all program administrators in the United States during the 1960's as they confronted the Joint Commission on Mental Illness and Health's challenge to design therapeutic and accessible psychiatric services. Central to the charting of new community mental health directions was the dilemma of whether to incorporate or redeploy the vast resources long expended for mental hospital programs. Few states could avoid this issue since for many decades the psychiatric system's services and personnel were controlled by these institutions. Mental hospitals had long been the community's bulwark against mental illness and represented society's preferred method of defending itself against the behaviorally deviant. However, the community mental health movement of the 1960's imposed a new belief system upon the thinking of citizens and professionals alike; in Chapter 3 we have presented our view of community mental health ideology's conceptual principles and operational practices. Could a mental hospital system composed of long isolated and custodially oriented facilities regain its viability by assuming contemporary mental health functions, or was this organizational system an anachronistic relic best disbanded and closed down?

Our analysis of this question is based upon the premise that a community mental health program's success or failure is not determined by any single factor, but rather by a complex interweaving of such variables as shifting ideologies, fluctuating organizational capacity and leadership, evolving personnel roles, expanded client expectations, the availability of alternative human services, etc. Accepting this approach to the study of program change, how can all of these multiple strands be woven into a cohesive theoretical framework capable of explaining the developments of the past decade?

Prior to the start of our research work in 1965, the available precedents for the comprehensive study of mental health program change can be categorized as falling within either the sociological process model or the goal attainment model. The former primarily emphasizes human relations concerns and intra-organizational processes, assuming that the key to major problems lies in the analysis of internal structure and functions. The works of Stanton and Schwartz (1954), Caudill (1958), and Goffman (1962) are excellent examples of the sophisticated analyses which emerged from the sociological process model. However, this model gives minimal consideration to quantitative measures of the program's operation. The influence of the environment is largely ignored, as are such other significant variables as the availability of people, technology, and money.

The goal attainment model for studying program change assumes that organizations are designed and operated to achieve specific predetermined objectives. By extending research techniques developed in the experimental laboratory into natural social settings, the model determines whether goals and objectives are attained. Such studies have been frequently conducted within psychiatric facilities, e.g., Ullmann's (1967) analysis of the Veterans Administration Hospital's effectiveness in discharging newly admitted patients. A major difficulty with this research model lies in the need to identify the independent variable or "cause" of an effect. As we undertook to study whether a mental hospital could assume community mental health responsibilities, it soon became evident that organizational effectiveness was not dependent upon the impact of any one variable or cause. Rather, the same outcome could be attained by manipulating differing initial conditions in varying ways. For example, a reduced inpatient census could be achieved by limiting new admissions and/or discharging chronic patients, depending upon staff and community receptivity to these strategies.

Recognizing the limitations of existing evaluative precedents, we considered it essential that any conceptual model to be employed in studying the changing mental hospital has to link the major variables of the organization's internal functioning, as well as account for the interrelations of the hospital and its community. The study of the hospital's role as a community mental health center requires simultaneous analysis of intra-organizational, extra-organizational, and inter-organizational processes. We have attempted to accomplish this aim, through the application of open systems concepts, whose variables and foci are presented in Chapter 4.

The open systems perspective is deemed particularly relevant to the study of mental hospital change since it generates meaningful constructs about the relationship of key variables to actions within the organization, while simultaneously considering an organization's interaction with its environment. We must emphasize, however, that open systems concepts are so broadranging and powerful in their data collecting and analytic requirements that we have more successfully utilized them for heuristic purposes than for direction of our day-to-day research activities. Thus, although the reader should view the open systems approach described in Chapter 4 as the theoretic framework within which we conducted our study of mental hospital change, he should not expect to find all of its analytical and methodological demands fulfilled in this report. Since our work is one of the first open systems studies of mental health organizations, we present it as a model for others to build upon and refine rather than as the definitive depiction of program change using an open systems approach.

The wisdom and utility of national and state mental health planning efforts, such as those described in Section I, must inevitably be tested at the local level; well-intentioned policies should be translatable into meaningful programs serving those in distress. Section II of our book focuses upon the efforts of Boston State Hospital, as an example of a large, prominent public psychiatric institution, to realign its traditional programmatic activities with the new community mental health mandate assigned to state mental hospitals by the Massachusetts Legislature. It should be noted that with regard to our work at Boston State Hospital, both authors acted as nonparticipant observers rather than as change agents or interventionists throughout their five-year study of this organization. This was the mutually agreed upon role that the authors negotiated with the hospital administration from the beginning of the research, and it was maintained throughout the study.

Chapters 5–9 focus upon the intra-, inter- and extraorganizational factors associated with a mental hospital's new program directions, and Chapter 10 considers the impact of these developments upon patient care. Since administrative and clinical structures appropriate to a broad array of community mental health functions differ significantly from those relevant to inpatient-focused services, Chapters 5 and 6 detail the manner whereby the unit system, a favorite form of mental hospital decentralization, is designed and implemented. The relationship of staff's ideological predilections and quest for modified professional roles to the hospital's structural and functional changes are explored in Chapters 7 and 8. A key challenge to the community-oriented mental hospital is that of establishing working linkages to the multiple environmental networks affecting its services. The inducements, constraints and systemic reverberations of doing so are presented in Chapter 9.

More effective clinical services and improved patient outcome are the fundamental purposes of the previously described organizational changes. In Chapter 10 we consider the impact of unitization and program modifications upon the care received by Boston State Hospital's patients at different points in time. This analysis is presented in open systems terms by focusing upon the hospital's growing efforts to utilize somatic clinical technologies for treating the community's inputs of disturbed persons. The hospital's patient outputs and the subsequent adjustments of discharged persons are also reviewed in Chapter 10.

Our study of mental hospital program change was initiated in 1965 within the still emerging parameters of community mental health ideology. However, events and experiences have unfolded so rapidly during the ensuing years that we find it necessary to close our book upon the disconcerting note that while many citizens and professionals still are grappling with the conceptual and practical implications of community mental health ideology, those on the cutting edge of service delivery already are refining the belief system of "human services." Section III presents our view of the conceptual and operational principles underlying efforts to expand the mental health professional's scope of concern even further during the 1970's. The ever more complex organizational networks required to insure comprehensive continuity of care for meeting diverse client needs are also cited in this final section.

The rapid shift from community mental health to human services ideology and the accelerated quest for more cohesive caregiving systems have been dizzying in their pace. Nevertheless, we must take pause and analyze their implications for the mental hospital as a contemporary caregiving organization. Have these large institutions successfully adapted to the demands of the community mental health era and, consequently, are they ready to undertake new human services activities as well? Or do mental hospitals, still functioning as archaic facilities primarily oriented to the inpatient custodial services of the past, finally need to be phased out? These questions pose the same profound and complex implications for the human services planner of the mid-1970's as they did for the community mental health planner in the mid-1960's. Chapter 11 describes some initial efforts to resolve them and suggests criteria for decisions incorporating patient care concerns as well as staff and community needs.

Acknowledgments

The authors accept responsibility for this book's premises, findings, and conclusions. Credit for its contributions must be shared, however, with the large number of individuals who have influenced our thinking and facilitated our work. The concepts of community mental health and human services which permeate our work were refined through stimulating discussions over many years with our mentors and colleagues—Dr. Gerald Caplan, Professor of Psychiatry, Harvard Medical School and Director of the Laboratory of Community Psychiatry; and Dr. Harold W. Demone, Jr., Associate Clinical Professor of Social Welfare, Harvard Medical School and Executive Vice President, United Community Planning Corporation. The research conducted at Boston State Hospital between 1965 and 1970 was only possible because of the unique cooperation and encouragement provided us by the Hospital's full staff, and particularly by its superintendents during this period, Drs. Milton Greenblatt and Jonathan Cole. The candor and receptivity to inquiry displayed by these two administrators were exemplary. A professional and administrative support staff of more than two dozen persons participated in our work for varying lengths of time, but space does not permit the listing of all their names. We would be remiss, however, to not publicly thank Mary Randall, Joanne Marks, and Greta Wheeler for their professional contributions, and Marguerite Slattery and Ericka Stackhouse for their invaluable secretarial assistance. Fiscal support for our work was provided by NIMH Grants MH-09214, MH-18382, and MH-13318 to the Laboratory of Community Psychiatry, Harvard Medical School. Dr. Howard Davis, Chief, Mental Health Services, Research and Development Branch, NIMH deserves special recognition for his constructive comments and invaluable help at various points in our work. Finally, a word of sincere appreciation to our wives and children who cheerfully encouraged us to persevere in this extended enterprise.

HCS and FB

Section I

Community Mental Health and Mental Hospitals

1. *Planning for Community Mental Health Programs*

An understanding of the manner in which the 1970s have come to emphasize human services delivery systems is greatly enhanced by comprehending their historical roots in the conception and design of community mental health programs a decade earlier. Although this particular thread was surely but one strand in the broader fabric of humanitarian concerns which dominated our society in the 1960s, community mental health concepts and techniques have singularly contributed to contemporary approaches for meeting citizens' human services needs. Thus, it is meaningful to open our analysis of evolving program trends by reviewing the aspirations, parameters and processes guiding community mental health planning efforts in the 1960s. This background is not only central to understanding the successes and failures of the subsequent decade, particularly as it affected mental hospitals, but also contains significant implications for the future.

HISTORICAL BACKGROUND

The period 1963–1965 was unprecedented in the mental health field, since it was the first time that nationwide activity had been undertaken to plan new programs which would redirect institutional patterns of care for the mentally ill into progressive community-based services. During this two-year period, official planning bodies in all 50 states engaged in intensive analyses of public and voluntary programs. These efforts culminated in comprehensive reports about the manner in which community mental health programs should be organized and administered, reports which formed the core of the plan submitted by each state to the National Institute of Mental Health for receipt of funds under the 1963 Community Mental Health Centers Act. For most states, these planning activities represented a unique opportunity to systematically analyze existing programs and to involve representative community professionals and nonprofessionals in designing program models and future priorities.

The nature of the planning activities, the types of procedures followed by planning bodies and the gamut of problems encountered by them were the most recent in a long series of program developments which had begun early this century, but did not fully crystallize until 1946 when Congress passed the National Mental Health Act. This legislation authorized a threefold program of research, training and service activities, and in 1948 the National Institute of Mental Health was established to administer and guide this program. A major milestone was reached in 1955 when Congress, through the Mental Health Study Act, authorized the Joint Commission on Mental Illness and Health to conduct a nationwide analysis and reevaluation of the human and economic problems of mental illness. On December 31, 1960, the Joint Commission transmitted its report, *Action for Mental Health*, to Congress, and it detailed a variety of recommendations. Of greatest relevance to this review was the Joint Commission's urging that the treatment of mental illness be reintegrated into the mainstream of community programming.

One specific outcome of the Joint Commission's report was that in January 1961 the Surgeon General's Ad Hoc

Committee on Planning Mental Health Facilities recommended "that the Governor of each state consider taking whatever steps are necessary to stimulate the development of a plan for mental health facilities [HEW, 1961]." Both the Conference of State and Territorial Mental Health Authorities, and the Governor's Conference, passed resolutions in 1962 strongly urging allocation of funds to enable development of comprehensive state planning efforts.

In response to the recommendations of these powerful groups, and the deep interest evidenced by President Kennedy in problems of mental illness and retardation, the 87th Congress appropriated $4.2 million in the 1963 NIMH budget. This was to be used for grant-in-aid to states for financing comprehensive mental health planning at the state level. Based upon a grant-in-aid formula, every state in the country was awarded a grant ranging from $50,000 to $280,000 for each of the two years to carry out the purposes of the planning program (HEW, 1963a).

As defined in the guidelines developed by NIMH (HEW, 1963b), the planning projects were specifically intended to improve the mental health of the people by developing community-based programs. These programs would provide a broad spectrum of mental health services by emphasizing a continuum of care and coordinating all relevant community resources. The goal of community-based programs was clearly imposed by NIMH. However, NIMH recognized that wide latitude would be necessary in achieving this goal because of differences among the states, their problems and resources, history and administrative structure

A second stipulation clearly imposed by the NIMH planning guidelines was that the state planning authority actively involve all appropriate agencies—public, private and voluntary. This stipulation is of major significance since it compelled the state mental health authority f purposes of planning, to involve all resources in the community functioning directly and indirectly in the area of mental health. The planning of community mental health programs, therefore, encompassed not only the thinking of the mental health professions but also that of the broad field of health and social welfare. It was clear, then, that the provision of comprehensive mental health services ranged beyond the psychiatric domain alone and would have to encompass those elements now commonly included within the rubric of human services.

THE PLANNING PROCESS

The process of planning for community mental health programs varied from state to state, but it is clear that similar problems and issues were encountered throughout the country as those concerned with community-oriented programs grappled with forces seeking to maintain the status quo (Glasscote & Kanno, 1963). The complexities of planning and the nature of those policy and program compromises required in our pluralistic society will be illustrated through a selective review of the issues encountered by Massachusetts's mental health planners (Schulberg, 1965; Schulberg, 1966a; Schulberg & Demone, 1966; Fogelson & Demone, 1969).

1. The Planner's Sanctions. The planner's ability to affect a caregiving network which includes diverse public, voluntary and private components very much depends upon the manner in which these audiences perceive his commitments and sanctions. To the degree that he is viewed as beholden to the interests of limited sectors, so will his ability to achieve broad-ranging solutions be constrained. The design of comprehensive mental health programs requires that the planner accommodate the needs of strong vested-interest groups, be sensitive to their unique concerns, and yet recognize the rights of competing interests. For example, if medical societies were accommodated in their desire to maintain the private-practice model as the program core, the planner risked failure in meeting the psychiatric interests of low-income and welfare clients (Schulberg, 1966b). Similarly, the support of citizen groups seeking to insure lay control over program development often could only be gained by the planner at the price of alienating professionals unaccustomed to sharing power. Consequently, the planner's actions would be divisive or fruitless unless he could counter dissent on a given issue with support from the widest possible range of political, professional and citizen groups.

2. *Flexible Coalitions.* Community mental health programs are sufficiently diverse to incorporate multiple policy positions and administrative practices. The planner's challenge is that of establishing flexible support coalitions for the program's numerous components so that opposition by a given group to specific elements will not endanger the community's support for the total effort. Thus, professional and citizen groups could agree on the fundamental concept of emphasizing community rather than institutionally based services while disagreeing on the locus of program control. Similarly, many psychiatrists and psychologists achieved consensus on the need to emphasize preventive services but disagreed as to whether nonphysicians could function effectively as program administrators. The planner's ability to juggle diverse power-interests on given issues while maintaining the total program balance is crucial to his success. Nevertheless, flexible coalitions with changing participants are highly fragile. They quickly dissolve in the face

of shifting pressures and priorities, and the planner must constantly build anew if his efforts are to remain viable.

3. Priority-Setting. An intrinsic aspect of program planning is the establishment of priorities for the use of scarce financial and manpower resources. Priorities can be determined by cataloguing the existing services available under both private and public auspices, gaining an indication of what are the most unmet needs, and analyzing the demographic and ecological characteristics of the areas to be be served. This information can be assembled by use of quantitative and qualitative indices which are generally available from primary and secondary sources. Having performed this effort, the planner must then come to grips with several constraints upon his decisions.

First, how valid are the data which he has assembled? The federal regulations for mental health planning had indicated that needs should be determined on the basis of the extent of mental illness and social pathology, socioeconomic indicators and welfare indices. Schulberg & Wechsler's (1967) analysis of these variables concluded that although they are interrelated to varying degrees, each is still sufficiently unique to warrant inclusion when assessing an area's need for multifaceted mental health services. Perhaps most significantly, consideration of environmental factors together with person-oriented indices casts mental health priority-setting into a broader framework than that traditionally used.

Having acknowledged the merits of an objective, data-oriented approach to priority-setting, the planner must recognize the influence of many "nonrational" factors. Demone (1965) has emphasized the extent to which crucial program-decisions are made outside of the mental health system by legislators and public administrators;

even the selection of goals is limited to certain choices, and they are value-laden with unanticipated or unintended consequences. Emphasizing these influences upon priority-setting is not intended to decry reason or to be nihilistic; but rather it is to encourage reality-testing through clear awareness of all forces at play. Thus, the planner pledged to data-based, objective criteria must temper his decisions with other inputs as well. For example, although a community's greatest need may be for children's services, adult programs may receive a higher priority if the latter have greater political support and/or are more easily funded. The planner's skill in balancing rational and nonrational concerns is crucial in determining priorities and fostering program development since the frequently antithetical nature of these concerns may produce controversial decisions with long-term consequences.

Many other dilemmas in addition to the previous three confronted mental health planners in their quest to establish broadly supported community mental health services. Despite a variety of pitfalls, most succeeded during the period 1963–1965 in formulating recommendations which would guide program development during the coming decade. Some recommendations were reaffirmations of previous thinking, but many others constituted an attempt to strike out in bold new directions.

The following principles were broadly accepted as basic to new undertakings: first, the patient must be the focus of a multifaceted program designed to meet his current needs; the patient must not be fitted into an institution's administrative needs. Second, a community mental health program must be comprehensive. It should include the five essential elements of inpatient, outpatient, emergency and partial hospitalization services, and education and consultation services. The program must serve all age groups, and especially those unable to afford private care. Third, continuity of care must be provided from the beginning to the end of psychiatric intervention. Private practitioners have long adhered to this principle, and it should be incorporated into organizational practice as well.

The Next Steps

Widespread hope was raised by the planning goals of establishing community mental health programs in which patients stay at home, are treated at home, and become well at home. If these goals were to be achieved, limited resources would have to be redeployed and the citizen's role in program planning and implementation would have to be reconsidered.

In most areas of any state, a comprehensive mental health program requires the coordination of multiple resources. To be truly effective, major and minor realignments of agency relationships would have to be negotiated. In the past, mental health and nonmental health agencies generally had interacted more by chance than through any mutual recognition of the benefits that planned cooperation could produce. As mental health programs assumed responsibility for serving all community residents, the collaboration of additional resources would be crucial. For example, the mental disorders of lower socioeconomic groups are so intertwined with real social problems that only rarely can they be solved through the skills of the psychiatrist alone. It was conceivable that the mental health problems of these groups would be the responsibility of agencies such as the welfare department, visiting nurses and community centers, in which event the mental health professional's primary role would be that of offering consultation, training and additional types of support rather than direct clinical services. The mental health center, then, would utilize fewer resources for patient care and more for indirect services like consultation and community organization.

Given the program goal of local inpatient units in all communities and in an effort to avoid duplicating scarce medical resources, it was likely that many community mental health programs would affiliate with the local general hospital. This arrangement would also permit the private practitioner to play a more active role in his patient's hospital care than had previously been possible.

The manner in which existing mental hospitals would be utilized in community-oriented programs constituted one of the most profound and controversial challenges to comprehensive planning. Advocates of federally funded community mental health programs asserted that the program's purposes included replacement of the existing mental hospital system with an alternative system which would provide services more effectively and reduce iatrogenic chronicity. However, as Chu & Trotter (1972) ruefully noted several years later, the NIMH regulations (HEW, 1964) for community mental health centers "prescribed no plans, mechanisms, nor procedures to guide centers in determining their relationship to state hospitals, no methods to divert potential state hospital admissions instead to community mental health centers, and no procedures whereby patients released from state hospitals could be rehabilitated and assisted back into the community. Indeed, the regulations contain not a single reference to the goal of supplanting state hospitals! This omission reveals perhaps the most erroneous set of assumptions underlying the community mental health centers program [Chu & Trotter, 1972, p. 12]."

Although this omission may retrospectively be lamentable, in the context of program needs in the mid-1960s, supplanting mental hospitals was not an entirely feasible goal. Planners clearly recognized that federal funds could support but a small segment of the vast resources required for comprehensive community mental health services, and that existing resources would have to be used as creatively as possible. Within this framework of practicality and optimism regarding the ability of anachronistic facilities to become contemporaneous, many planners viewed a mental hospital as serving two distinct purposes. The first is the provision of the five essential services in a comprehensive mental health program to the geographic area in which it is located. This would be possible when new local inpatient programs relieved mental hospitals of much of their current admission loads. The second purpose of a mental hospital would be to provide continued treatment facilities for its own local area as well as for neighboring community mental health programs.

It would be important to facilitate the free movement of patients between outpatient clinics, acute inpatient services and continued care facilities. In those instances where a mental hospital provided continued care for several community programs, the hospital might well consider establishing a geographic unit system on the continued treatment service as one way of facilitating two-way communication and transfer of patients with local centers. When geographical distance is not an issue, the state hospital and its neighboring community mental health centers could experiment with an arrangement whereby each center is responsible, or participates, in the professional staffing of its unit.

Citizen Participation

Planners recognized that the goal of statewide community mental health centers would not be achieved within a brief period of time but was rather a goal to be pursued over the coming decade. A phasing process would be necessary, and the speed of implementation would depend upon such factors as the availability of fiscal support, the recruitment of manpower, and citizen interest and participation. This last element contained many problematic features and subtle nuances which to this day have remained controversial as citizens and professionals grope to clarify their respective roles and responsibilities.

It should be noted that the idea of citizen volunteers and local participation in the shaping and operating of community programs is not a radical one. Public welfare boards, public health boards, public school committees and the federal requirement of citizen participation in urban renewal and poverty programs are based upon this concept. The mental health field, although relatively recent in its development, is no exception to recognizing the merits of this approach. In fact, mental health planning projects exerted considerable effort to insure the participation of key citizen groups in program reviews and in the formulation of future plans. Public hearings at which local spokesmen could discuss the impact of new proposals were commonplace.

The nature of ongoing citizen participation, however, raised different power and program issues. Proposals for citizen input ranged from those advocating administrative structures in which citizens would have decisionmaking authority to those which would restrict citizens to purely advisory roles. Furthermore, it was quite evident that citizen interest and concern tended to focus more on the newly evolving community-based services than on the existing institutionally based ones. The potential glamour of community mental health programs far outshone the shadowy image of mental hospitals, and citizen interest obviously was attracted to the former rather than the latter programs. Nevertheless, effective community program development required citizen concern and commitment to all of the community's resources and the planner was challenged to insure that this did indeed occur.

SUMMARY

The period of 1963 to 1965 was one in which an almost evangelistic fervor developed among this country's mental health interests as the promise of a bold new approach to the care of the mentally ill loomed brightly on the horizon. Statewide planning projects had generated considerable enthusiasm among professionals and citizens for new program undertakings, and the future was being approached with unbridled optimism. Federal funds for the construction and staffing of community mental health centers represented an attractive carrot potentially capable of generating system change far beyond that of their absolute dollar amount.

Mental health planners recognized that despite the previous poor ability of mental hospitals to offer quality services to their patients, mental hospitals, nevertheless, controlled significant resources. The fundamental dilemma was whether these physical and manpower resources could be constructively molded into progressive caregiving programs, or whether the mental hospital as an organization had to be dismantled. Within the planning constraints of 1965, the first choice was one of high risk but also one with high potential dividends. The second choice appealed to those with a revolutionary spirit but was deemed by many planners to be highly impractical in terms of contemporary options.

The remainder of this book is concerned with the interwoven foci of evolving community mental health and human services program concepts, and the attempt of mental hospitals to function within these contemporary parameters. The organizational consequences of mandating the mental hospital to join the mainstream of program development in the 1960s and 1970s will be analyzed within the framework of open systems concepts, reflecting our belief that the modern psychiatric institution is affected by a variety of external and internal influences which interact in complex ways.

2. *The Prospective Role of the Mental Hospital*

The burgeoning community mental health programs of the mid-1960s sprouted in many directions and assumed varied organizational and service characteristics. One significant pattern involved the efforts of traditional mental hospitals to shed anachronistic organizational structures and clinical responsibilities so as to become contemporary in structure and function. This process did not occur in a vacuum; instead, it occurred within a time frame and a sociological matrix influenced by and dependent upon several disparate factors. The change process was affected by distant and immediate historical events such as those described earlier, as well as by the future needs of the institution's social environment. The institution's unique organizational history and contemporary goals were similarly significant in determining the nature of change. Finally, since the community-oriented mental hospital is, by definition, a component of a larger network of caregiving resources, its change process must be understood as affecting and being affected by the caregiving system of which it is a part. This chapter outlines the complexity of the organizational and environmental forces which abetted, as well as constrained, the mental hospital of the mid-1960s in its struggle to assume a new role, to incorporate new functions, and to respond to new demands as it entered the era of community mental health. We shall especially consider the concept "community mental health" because of its multiple implications for the mental hospital in transition.

THE RISE AND FALL OF THE MENTAL HOSPITAL

A historical review of the mental hospital's role in providing psychiatric services reveals both the best and the worst in our treatment of the mentally ill. Even more important, it strikingly indicates that the position of the mental hospital was not always an isolated one, and that for a period of time in the mid-nineteenth century, the mental hospital movement embodied the same societal goals which are now associated with community mental health programs. The Caplans (1969) describe the repeated attempts of early psychiatrists to join the lay and medical communities in promoting preventive measures, in attacking misconceptions about the mentally ill, and in trying to insure that the mentally ill would assume the normal social prerogatives of citizens. The idea that environment has a major influence in creating and curing mental insanity was also common in the mid-nineteenth century, and this led professionals to attempt to mold hospital and community milieus accordingly.

Grob (1966) indicates that when mental hospitals were first established in the early 1800s, therapy, not custodial care, was their primary function. It had become clear that the care of the indigent insane within the framework of the poor-laws was increasingly inadequate and that a medically supervised, more therapeutic approach was required. The results achieved by the treatment programs of some early mental hospitals were impressive even by modern standards. In 1841, Samuel Woodward, the first superintendent of Worcester State Hospital in Massachusetts, reported that in the first seven years of the hospital's operation, recovery rates among individuals insane for less than one year ranged between 82 and 91 percent (Grob, 1962). Equally significant is the fact that more than a century ago, Woodward already emphasized the need for early treatment, since recovery rates for individuals insane for more than one year only ranged between 16 and 23 percent.

The therapeutic programs of mental hospitals in the mid-nineteenth century were similar, in many ways, to those of a modern facility. Contemporary medications, particularly narcotics, were prescribed since insanity was thought of in somatic terms. It was also recognized, however, that a healthy psychological environment was essential in the treatment process, and moral therapy too became a cornerstone of the treatment program. In fact, the "therapeutic community" of modern times has many of its origins in the era of moral therapy which predominated in nineteenth-century American psychiatry (Bockoven, 1956).

The mental hospital achieved its greatest respect and effectiveness during the "moral" therapy period of approximately 1830 to 1850; however, during the 1850s decline set in. Descriptions of the mental hospital's subsequent ebb and flow appear in the mental health literature (Caplan & Caplan, 1969; Deutsch, 1948; Gorman, 1956; Grob, 1966). Among the factors producing decline was the failure of "scientific psychiatry"; instead, the mental hospital's development was determined predominantly by external and internal social, psychological, economic and intellectual influences. Moral treatment was not founded on systematic theory; rather, it developed out of the humanitarian and religious concepts of the period and was based upon a close relationship between patient and therapist both of whom had a common cultural heritage. However, as patients from diverse ethnic, religious and economic backgrounds entered the hospital, moral treatment became less and less successful.

The failure of moral therapy also led to the uncovering of the "myth of curability" (Caplan & Caplan, 1969). The claim of curing insanity had attracted active, idealistic men to the profession of psychiatry and induced the public to invest large sums on expensive facilities. Disillusionment with inflated claims of curability produced alienation among laymen, who questioned the wisdom and necessity of large expenditures for the insane, and among psychiatrists who doubted their personal efficacy as therapists. The Caplans point out the vicious circle which was thus created. The inability to cure patients, plus the flow of new cases, produced overcrowded conditions which, in turn, lowered professional effectiveness and resulted finally in an even greater backlog of chronic cases.

The degeneration of the mental hospital into a custodial institution in turn influenced psychiatric theory. Noting the reduced effectiveness of "moral" treatment, psychiatrists rejected the role of psychological factors and reverted to an emphasis on somaticism. However, as Grob (1966) points out, a strictly somatic approach usually led to therapeutic nihilism, which further transformed mental hospitals into vast holding operations; mentally ill patients were to be confined until that distant day when specific cures for specific disease-entities would become available.

If the mental hospital's existence could not be justified by the number of patients it cured, then its custodial function had to be emphasized. Inevitably, societal concerns and the hospital's orientation produced a situation in which support of the mental hospital was based on the rationale that it provided protection against groups menacing the safety and security of society. Legislative funding in the early 1900s was directed at providing accommodations to care for the growing number of chronically disturbed individuals. But, as the congressionally established Joint Commission on Mental Illness and Health (1961) trenchantly noted many years later, mental hospitals long have been the first public institutions to suffer in bad times and the last to benefit in good times. Deterioration accelerated during the Depression of the 1930s, and the financial setbacks of this period were subsequently compounded by the manpower shortages caused by World War II. New hospitals could not be built, and few old ones were repaired. Meager professional staffs were depleted further, and institutional morale reached its lowest point in fifty years.

The damage during the years of World War II to the care of the mentally ill, who were maintained in houses of horror, was well documented during the postwar period, and public and professional concern was rekindled. Deutsch (1948) described the snakepit conditions existing in mental hospitals near large metropolitan centers, and he emphasized the fact that not one single public mental hospital had ever met even the minimum standards set by the American Psychiatric Association in all major aspects of care and treatment. Subsequently, innovative therapeutic programs were undertaken in some public mental hospitals (Greenblatt, York, & Brown, 1955), and inpatient populations began to decline with the use of tranquilizers.

On the whole, however, public acceptance of and support for the improved mental hospital were not reflected in increased financial allocations. Many ambitious postwar programs for mental hospitals were dropped as budget retrenchments hit one state after another, and even apparent budget increases were eaten up by inflationary costs. Studies by the Joint Commission on Mental Illness and Health revealed that the average daily expenditure for patients in state, county and city mental hospitals by 1960 was still maintained at a custodial level of $4.44, as compared to the $27.65 per diem cost expended in state and local general hospitals for acute patient care. Further, the ratio of employees to patients was 2.1:1 in the general hospital but only 0.3:1 in the mental hospital. Thus, despite certain signs of progress in the 1950s, the Joint Commission concluded in 1961 that half of the patients in state hospitals received no active treatment of any kind designed to improve their mental condition. This situation applied particularly to patients on continued treatment wards, most of whom were found to be receiving no treatment at all.

Recommendations of Joint Commission on Mental Illness and Health

Faced with a congressional mandate to recommend a national program for the control of mental illness, the Joint Commission studies uncovered a variety of disparities between what needed to be done and what was actually being done. The Commission concluded that progress depended upon the solution of the longstanding problems of manpower, facilities and costs. Primarily concerned with the treatment of existing mental illness, the Commission recommended as an objective of a national mental health program that one fully staffed, full-time community mental health clinic be established for every 50,000 citizens. Such clinics would serve both adults and children and were to be regarded as the main agent in reducing the need for prolonged or repeated hospitalization. This recommendation was based on the conviction that mental disorders are best treated in the local community, preferably on an outpatient or day-care basis. Inpatient treatment, if necessary, was projected for a brief duration and was to be provided in the community either in the psychiatric unit of a general hospital or in a special psychiatric facility. Removal of the mentally ill to a distant hospital was viewed as a prime factor in producing chronicity and should be avoided if at all possible.

The recommended role of the mental hospital in a national program proved to be one of the most controversial aspects of the Joint Commission's report. A few years earlier, in his Presidential Address to the American Psychiatric Association, Harry Solomon (1958) had stated:

> The large mental hospital is antiquated, outmoded, and rapidly becoming obsolete . . . I do not see how any reasonably objective view of our mental hospitals today can fail to conclude that they are bankrupt beyond remedy. I believe, therefore, that our large mental hospitals should be liquidated as rapidly as possible in an orderly and progressive fashion [p. 7].

The Joint Commission agreed with this assessment. It urged that no new state hospitals of more than 1,000 beds be built and that not a single patient should be added to facilities already housing more than 1,000 patients. Furthermore, it suggested that all existing mental hospitals of more than 1,000 beds be gradually and progressively converted into centers for the longterm and combined care of chronic diseases, including mental illness. This proposal was based on the Commission's opinion that many of the facilities needed for the prolonged care of mental patients are identical with those needed for the continued care of any chronic physical illness; communities would, therefore, find it more practical to care for all chronic patients in the same hospital. The Joint Commission predicted that implementation of this proposal would encounter many realistic obstacles such as funding and administration, but emphasized that the major delay would come in getting people to look at the problem realistically and objectively.

The role of the smaller mental hospital was viewed differently by the Joint Commission. It recommended that facilities with 1,000 beds or less, suitably located for regional service, should be converted into intensive treatment centers. Patients with major mental illness in the acute stages, or chronic patients with a good prospect for recovery, could be properly treated at these facilities. The Commission noted that the most important requirement for an intensive treatment center is a well-trained and competent staff at least as large in number as the patients served. It also stressed that, with but few exceptions, psychiatric leadership would be necessary in the executive department if the hospital was to function as a therapeutic environment for patients.

Effects of the Community Mental Health Centers Act

The major recommendations of the Joint Commission were ultimately incorporated in the 1963 Community Mental Health Centers Act (Public Law 88-164) whereby Congress authorized federal assistance for the construction of centers which would provide at least the following five essential services for citizens residing within their geographic areas: inpatient and outpatient care, emergency services, partial hospitalization, and consultation and education. Among the goals envisioned for this program by President Kennedy was the reduction of the number of mental patients then under custodial care by 50 percent or more within a decade or two. It was clearly recognized, however, that while the new community centers were being developed, certain resources of the existing mental hospitals needed strengthening. President Kennedy, therefore, urged in his 1963 message to Congress that the federal government financially assist mental hospitals during the transition period to undertake demonstration and pilot projects, to improve the quality of care, and to provide in-service training for the personnel manning these institutions. As a result, Congress approved the Hospital Improvement Program, one goal of which was to integrate the individual institution's activities into an overall statewide program.

Despite this financial assistance to mental hospitals, it was clear that the major thrust of future federal support would be for community mental health centers. Considerable uncertainty, controversy and even acrimony arose among planners, administrators, and clinicians as to the future role of existing public mental hospitals. The reactions of mental hospital directors developed in several directions, some constructive, some destructive, still others simply expressing a plaintive plea for maintaining the status quo. Glass (1964) advised his colleagues that "there is no immediate problem. The difficulties of obtaining financial support and trained personnel are of such magnitude as to make inevitable a considerable delay in the establishment of the community program."

Glass, Hoch (1964) and others assembled various indices to support their contention that the mental hospital would always be needed in a comprehensive program. They noted that admissions to public mental hospitals continued to increase despite the continued growth of community clinics, psychiatric units in general hospitals, and private practitioners. Although the general population increased only 11 percent between 1956 and 1962, admissions to public mental hospitals rose 46 percent during that period. Hoch indicated that the release rate from New York mental hospitals had increased by 75 percent from 1955 to 1963, but in this same period admissions rose by 40 percent. With increasing public confidence in state hospitals and the effectiveness of their treatment programs, Hoch concluded that mental hospitals were and would continue treating more patients than ever before in their history.

The role of the mental hospital in serving the chronically ill was generally acknowledged by all. Hoch (1964) stressed that a hard core of schizophrenic and organically ill patients would remain, who would continue to require the services of the large mental hospital. Although the responsibility for the chronically mentally ill would remain with the hospitals, it remained unclear how they could best care for them. The Joint Commission had recommended that a chronic disease center must emphasize rehabilitation services and that it could be operated by a trained administrator, layman or physician, with psychiatrists providing necessary consultation. Despite the fact that new approaches plainly seemed warranted and that psychiatry's record with these patients was far from admirable, O'Neill (1960) argued that "the chronic mental patient is a medical responsibility and I am sure that American psychiatry will not abandon him to the care of educators, public health persons, sociologists, or city planners [p. 813]."

In general, then, supporters of mental hospitals were contending that these facilities would continue to be needed for several reasons. In many instances, the newly developed community resources were serving as excellent casefinders and creating a fresh demand for mental hospital services. In other instances, community facilities and mental hospitals would operate as two separate systems, each serving a population which differed in severity of symptoms, clinical course and socioeconomic status. It was thought that many types of patients (including antisocial individuals, those exhibiting bizarre behavior, the seriously depressed and suicidal and those lacking family support) are simply not suitable for community care and would continue to require the services of the mental hospital. Finally, even with the rapid development of community facilities, certain other trends, such as increased patient longevity, were thought to be reversing the decline of mental hospital populations and creating new need for these facilities.

As is often the case in the formulation of comprehensive health plans, fanciful theoretical arguments about the mental hospital's future role yielded to the exigencies of financing, manpower and politics. After the initial sense of satisfaction over passage of Public Law 88-164 abated, it became evident that the federal construction and staffing funds would provide little more than seed money. In states requiring many new centers, the initial federal funds would be sufficient to construct only a few.

Given this realization, the role of existing mental hospitals was reappraised by those responsible for comprehensive program development. Since the bulk of necessary construction and operating funds would continue to come from local and state budgets, most states concluded that a viable network of community mental health resources would require the mental hospital as an integral component. It also became evident that these facilities were no longer as geographically isolated as they had been in the past. The combination of metropolitan expansion and growing transportation networks had reduced the physical and psychological distance of the hospital from its community.

The early community mental health acts passed in the 1950s by such big states as New York and California accentuated the mental hospital's role as a continuing-care facility with little direct involvement in preventive intervention or intensive treatment. By 1965, however, states could no longer afford to disregard the mental hospital's potential for serving as the core of certain comprehensive programs, and new plans were formulated accordingly. The Massachusetts Mental Health Planning Project (1965), for example, recommended that within a statewide comprehensive program the mental hospital be viewed as serving two distinct purposes: (1) providing the five essential services in a comprehensive program to the immediate geographic area in which it is located; and (2) providing continued treatment facilities for its own area as well as for several contiguous communities.

The focus of planners and program directors had shifted, then, from viewing the mental hospital as a primarily custodial facility, and consideration was being given to ways in which the hospital could be updated and revamped so that it would function effectively as a comprehensive center. Various suggestions for change were made (e.g., Glass, 1964; Levy, 1965), but they essentially centered around four major themes.

1. A treatment orientation. The structure, administration and services of the mental hospital should be oriented to the single purpose of meeting a patient's therapeutic needs. Of particular importance would be the speedy elimination of dehumanizing conditions of patient care.

2. Flexible treatment programs. Patients should not be forced to fit the mold of dysfunctional treatment patterns, but rather treatment patterns should be adapted to the patient's needs. Day and night hospitals are highly desirable for the acutely ill, while vocational rehabilitation services are essential for the chronically ill. Continuity of care should have the highest priority in revised treatment efforts.

3. Reducing the hard-core population. In most institutions more than 50 percent of the patient population had been hospitalized for several years, creating a severe drain on limited resources. The resulting custodial orientation could be reversed if facilities set the goal of achieving a 1:1 staff-patient ratio, possibly through reorganizing clinical services into semiautonomous units.

4. A community orientation. The mental hospital should no longer function as a self-contained entity responsive only to its own needs but must instead be prepared constantly to interact with its environment. Clinical units organized on the basis of geographic catchment areas constitute a possible administrative structure which would permit professional staff and community members to develop productive relationships.

COMMUNITY MENTAL HEALTH CONCEPTS

A meaningful analysis of the ways in which mental hospitals have moved to exercise their revitalized franchise in the era of community mental health requires a clear understanding of the concepts, ideologies and values prevalent during these years. In our viewpoint, community mental health is the most recent in a long series of psychiatric ideologies or belief systems which affect the theoretical foundations and design of mental health caregiving networks (Baker & Schulberg, 1967; Schulberg & Baker, 1969). Clearly validated etiological models of mental illness are as sparse today as a century ago, and practitioners are forced to function on the basis of psychiatric belief systems which are compatible with their view of the relationship between man, pathological forces and the illness process.

The specific strands which have contributed to the development of community mental health ideology were traced by Caplan & Caplan (1966). It is clear that the current belief system did not arise *de nouveau* but, rather, incorporates both philosophies and activities dating back many decades in addition to concepts of much more recent vintage. Advances in the somatic and psychotherapeutic approaches to mental illness have been intertwined with a growing recognition of the need to modify pathological environmental influences. Comprehensive programs of prevention, treatment and aftercare were described as early as 1909 by Adolph Meyer, but for many years momentum for community-oriented concepts could not be sustained. Not until after World War II were some of the gaps which had weakened the earlier mental hygiene movement filled through research, new services and broadened public support. Only then did we witness advances in mental hospital practices, a concern with community services and a growth in governmental financing for mental health services.

Although the 1964 federal guidelines defining the nature of community mental health programs would appear to be straightforward, these guidelines have been the subject of widely varying interpretation. At one pole are those who contend that the minimally required services of a community mental health program are those which progressive hospitals have been providing for some time, and the new term is but a euphemism for existing activities. To those at the other pole, however, the integration of clinical services into a comprehensive program certainly represents great progress, but they put even more emphasis on the key role the program must play in initiating necessary social and political reform through consultation and education. Since most mental health personnel profess general support for the community mental health approach, it is necessary to recognize that the specific program directions which they emphasize are related to a view of the etiology and treatment of mental illness. Three related and yet significantly differing frameworks have loomed prominent.

The first and most commonly followed conceptual framework defines pathology as being primarily intrapsychic, i.e. occurring in individual patients. This approach has much in common with the *medical model of illness* in which the etiologic cause may be an environmental agent, e.g., a virus, or an experience of deprivation, but the agent is viewed as initiating processes within the individual himself, culminating in illness. Rather than attacking the offending agent before it can impair its victim, the treatment strategy of this medical-like model usually consists of nullifying or removing the pathogenic agent through the use of drugs, or by interventions such as psychotherapy and rehabilitation programs, so that restorative forces within the individual can bring about recovery.

Many classic as well as recent treatment techniques fall well within this framework. The psychoanalytic approach focuses upon the individual's dynamic conflicts and helps him bring repressed materials into consciousness so that healthier behavior patterns may emerge. Short-term or time-limited psychotherapy is a recent modification of this technique intended to shorten the duration of treatment, but essentially it too is based upon an intrapsychic conception of pathology. The widely heralded crisis-intervention techniques flow from this framework as well, since they are based upon the rationale that, during a crisis situation, the patient's personality structure is in a state of flux, his defences are less rigid and his behavior is more amenable to change. There is no intention of altering the patient's basic intrapsychic personality structure, but it is hoped that the aggregate of psychological forces producing disturbed behavior can be brought into better equilibrium through well-timed interventions. Finally, the various behavior-therapy techniques receiving increased attention among psychologists are directed at the individual's intrapsychic structure, as well as upon the premise that he has developed maladaptive behavior patterns which can be modified under proper learning conditions. The emphasis, again, is upon intervening at the point where the individual's intrapsychic disturbance has reached a level which necessitates external assistance.

The services emanating from the intrapsychic conception of mental illness generally have been of high quality. However, they can assist only a few of those requiring help. Therefore, the general public has become increasingly dissatisfied with the relatively small contribution made by facilities utilizing this approach toward reducing the community's overall burden. Consequently, there has been a greater willingness among mental health professionals to adopt the public health model as a guide for enlarging their scope of concern.

Under the *public health model*, the community mental health worker not only accepts responsibility for his individual patients but is also concerned with the needs of the total population. The population may be defined in terms of geographically bounded areas like a city or neighborhood, or in functional terms, such as a student body, a trade union or the armed services. The population approach assimilates the medical model of illness in that pathology can still be considered an internal phenomenon, but greater recognition often is given to environmental factors. It differs in that the public health practitioner also views casefinding and prevention as appropriate activities in addition to the diagnostic and treatment functions of the practitioner in the medical-like model.

The third conceptual framework may be called the *problems-in-living model*. It is markedly different in structure and implications from the individual-oriented framework noted above. Illness is no longer perceived as an entirely intrapsychic process, but rather as a disequilibrium between certain individuals and their environment. This model focuses on the social structure of a community as an interlocking network of roles which are occupied by individual members, each of whom is expected to perform tasks and to receive privileges commensurate with his place in society. From this perspective, individual symptoms do not reflect internal pathology but rather an impairment in the individual's ability to assume a proper role and develop satisfactory relationships with others. The implications of this socially oriented framework change the traditional boundaries of the mental health professional's functions quite radically, particularly when contrasted with those of colleagues who focus on the intrapersonal dynamics of individual patients. Because of this concern with the relationship of environments to the welfare of total populations, it becomes especially necessary for the mental health professional to engage in activities of a preventive nature.

Each of the three models guiding community mental health developments contains novel as well as familiar implications for mental hospital programs. It is important to stress again that community mental health ideology is not totally new but rather embodies concepts which have long guided as well as troubled mental hospital personnel. For many decades, the medical model of illness has been at the base of most treatment programs for psychotics, and this model has achieved its greatest relevance with the development of effective psychiatric drugs. The public health model, with its implication of responsibility for total populations, is familiar to the mental hospital since it traditionally has cared for all of its community's chronically ill as well as for many of those experiencing acute breakdowns. The problem-in-living framework, which stresses that maladjustment represents a disequilibrium between the individual and his environment, has guided mental hospital social therapy programs since the days of moral treatment, and is being utilized increasingly in the rehabilitation chronic patients.

CHANGING THE MENTAL HOSPITAL

In his review of "Action for Mental Health" at the 1963 Mental Hospital Institute, Smith (1964) stressed that the basic significance of the Joint Commission's report was its emphasis on the need for change in the mental hospital's goals and structures. The report had specified many of the new goals confronting psychiatric institutions, and challenged the organizations to experiment with new structures better suited to achieving the goals of the 1960s. In the decade since the Joint Commission's report, it has become abundantly clear that the mental hospital truly can become an integral component of comprehensive programs in those instances where the organizational challenge is met and change occurs.

Progress toward achieving new goals and developing revised clinical and administrative structures has occurred in various ways. Limited resources are being stretched further by reducing hard-core populations. A 1969 NIMH report indicated that there had been a 24 percent decrease between 1955 and 1967 in the number of patients in the year-end resident population of state and county mental hospitals. By early 1972 NIMH reported that in the four-year period 1967–1971 the inpatient population had declined an additional 28%. Furthermore, in 1968 mental hospitals accounted for only 25 percent of all patient-care episodes, in contrast to 1955 when they had accounted for 50 percent of all such episodes.

In addition to reduced populations, other changes are necessary if the goals and structure of the mental hospital are to be geared for active participation in a community mental health program. The three conceptual models described in the previous section imply different methods of defining the mental hospital's community, participating in the community's caregiving network, modifying its clinical and administrative technology and utilizing its professional and nonprofessional personnel. The remainder of this chapter will explore these tasks and approaches to their completion.

Definitions of Community

Perhaps no aspect of a community mental health program remains more ambiguous and troublesome than the boundaries of the geographic sector which it is to serve. The increased complexity of urban living patterns has led to the dissolution of natural communities within which implicit bonds related person to person, and within which the roles of community members were set by tradition and cultural expectation. Instead, today's dominant type of community leads people to relate to one another through formulated guidelines, or even rules and regulations. Major blocks of time are spent in formal institutions like places of employment and civic organizations rather than in home neighborhoods. Panzetta (1971) has contended that community psychiatrists erroneously have sought to establish programs based upon their longing for the traditional "gemeinschafts" while failing to accept the reality of our contemporary "gesellschafts."

One approach to programming for our contemporary society is Demone & Schulberg's (1971) suggestion that a flexible "community of solution" be used for delineating areas within which human services care-systems can be organized and administered. The community of solution will vary according to program purposes. In some instances several small areas can be combined into a large region; for other purposes single small areas can stand independently. For example, a comprehensive health planning project's "community" should be large enough to include most service programs so that only rare medical problems need be serviced outside of the geographic region. A neighborhood health center's community, however, should be small enough so that all residents have ready access to the facility, and the area should contain few enough people so that staff can efficiently meet demands for emergency care, preventive activities, etc.

The 1964 NIMH regulations for implementing community mental health programs defined the "community of solution" simply as 75,000 to 200,000 people, leaving unspecified the modifications required by such factors as varying density levels, socioeconomic status, urban or rural location, extent of existing services, etc. The NIMH definition has created the least difficulty for mental hospitals whose services are based upon the medical model of illness. These facilities are primarily concerned with individuals already acutely or chronically ill and the specific geographic locations from which patients emanate generally have been of administrative rather than etiologic significance. Nevertheless, even mental hospitals which view pathology as intrapsychic or somatic must link their services with those of other community resources if continuity of care is to be provided. Developing necessary linkages often involves complex administrative considerations, and the congruence of geographic areas being served by relevant programs can significantly affect patient care.

The limitations of a geographic, administrative or quantitative definition of community have led some planners to espouse more psychological, ecological and sociological conceptions of the "community of solution." This approach is particularly relevant for those reorganizing mental hospitals on the basis of the problems-in-living model since it postulates an intimate relationship between an individual's adjustment and the nature of his environment. An ecological approach to determining the size and nature of the community was presented by Kelly (1966), who defined predictable patterns of individual behavior which are specific to given social situations. From this perspective, behavior is not viewed as sick or well but is defined as transactional—an outcome of reciprocal interactions between specific social situations and the individual. Klein (1968) and Lehmann (1971) have also proposed an interactional relationship between the individual and his environment which similarly highlights the significance of the community to the mental health of its population.

It is clear that the emphases placed upon the environment's role in triggering and treating mental illness affect both the definition of "community" and the responsibilities of the mental hospital staff member. Psychological, ecological and sociological conceptions suggest that the community-oriented mental hospital worker should actively promote environments appropriate to the emotional needs of local residents. To accomplish this, the staff must understand the local environment, become immersed in its dynamics and even function as social-change agents. Even within the medically oriented facility, however, the staff must also become involved in such unusual but vital tasks as determining how community decisions are made, funds allocated and new programs initiated and supported. The opportunities and hazards awaiting the professional venturing into the community have been clearly described by Caplan (1964), Howe (1964) and Shaw & Eagle (1971), who suggest strategies of approach for avoiding possible pitfalls.

The Caregiving Network

One of the most critical problems in effectively operating a community mental health program is the design of a caregiving network capable of providing the essential services. Regardless of which of the previously discussed conceptual models is employed, in many communities it is not feasible for a single facility to provide by itself all of the required services. Conversely, elements of the comprehensive program may already be provided by agencies other than the mental health center, and duplication would be both wasteful and harmful to interagency cooperation. Consensus, thus, has arisen about the need for mental health facilities to collaborate with other community resources, but there still is considerable controversy about the specific nature of such relationships. For purposes of describing the contrasting arrangements, they can be categorized as the medical organization network and the human services network (Schulberg, 1969). Since these caregiving networks are based upon differing conceptual models, they vary in their functional and administrative details. The medical organizational network, generally speaking, utilizes facilities whose services are based upon the medical conception of illness. The human services network is more likely to incorporate community caregiving facilities which pursue the problems-in-living approach. Various aspects of the public health conceptual model have been incorporated into both of these organizational networks.

The medical organizational network can be described as a caregiving arrangement in which the mental health center, under medical leadership, assumes responsibility and perhaps supervision of all the community's mental health services. The resources of other agencies are clearly seen as being of value but basically supportive in character. The program can be schematically represented as a circle at the center of which is a psychiatric facility. Around the periphery are the community agencies, each with different functions and goals. The mental health center's role is viewed as that of coordinator of existing services, innovator of new services, educator, administrator and consultant to the community.

Along with the medical organization network, increasing attention is being given to the human services network as an alternative administrative arrangement for organizing a community mental health program. A number of studies have shown that many nonpsychiatric community agencies function as mental health caregivers and that the mental health of a community is vitally affected by their services. Hence, the mental health center is viewed as only one of many community resources which cooperate to serve the mental health needs of all citizens. This network is especially evident in rural areas and in those areas where mental health programs have assumed a strong social action stance. The mental health facility and other agencies jointly work with the same troubled family, cooperate in the development of new programs and try to minimize competition with one another.

Each of these organizational networks provides the mental hospital with a different role. The medical organizational network is more suitable for the hospital which adheres to an intrapsychic model of illness and considers itself to be the community's primary resource for treating the mentally ill. The human services network provides a more effective framework for the mental hospital which has begun to consider itself responsible for citizens experiencing problems-in-living. Nevertheless, both networks feature a mental health program which is broadly based and which incorporates the resources of many facilities rather than being predominantly centered in any one. Greenblatt & Schulberg (1970) cite the following systems as ones with which an active, community-oriented mental hospital must develop effective linkages: government, citizen volunteers, education, professional organizations, research and development and caregivers. The effectiveness of comprehensive programs is, in this view, directly related to the coordinated effort of an interacting, linked network. For the network to be viable, it must be sensitive to the aspirations and limitations of its component members as well as being aware of the varied ways in which environmental forces influence it.

Technological Capabilities

It is fair to state that despite the major changes occurring in the ideological base of many existing psychiatric programs, relatively few advances are evident in the technology through which these new community-oriented programs are to be realized. Indeed, refinement of the concepts inherent in the community mental health belief system is far outstripping the technology needed to implement it. Lanyon (1971) contends that the mental health industry is essentially pretechnological because of the considerable resistance to formally identifying necessary skills, preferring the craftsman or artist mystique. To be sure, advocates of the community mental health approach have been active in developing such new techniques as crisis intervention, short-term therapy, consultation to caregivers, primary prevention services, etc., but the application of these techniques, particularly by mental hospitals, remains limited. Nevertheless, many institutions still contend that they are community mental health centers despite their use of primarily longterm, individually oriented treatment approaches, which are as limited in their community impact today as they were in previous decades.

The emphasis which community mental health ideology places upon comprehensive services to a specified population requires that we refine the technology of both our clinical techniques and the administrative patterns upon which services are organized. Loeb (1966) has described the spectrum of services necessary for insuring continuity of care as "levels of sustaining, each with its appropriate interventions and agencies of intervention [p. 227]." The spectrum begins and ends with the person's "intimates," and the objective of a community mental health program should be to minimize the intervention required from caregivers who assume fulltime responsibility for the individual, as in the total care provided by a mental hospital. A "linking" technique for achieving this new objective has been developed by Hansell (1968), and the thrust of both his model and that of Loeb is in devising new clinical technology and administrative management structures so that existing services can be better integrated and coordinated.

A review of the clinical technologies introduced into and utilized by mental hospitals during the past two decades shows that the major thrusts have been toward increased utilization of psychiatric drugs, refinement of social therapeutic and rehabilitation programs, and application of behavioral reinforcement procedures. Verbal therapy, of both an individual and group nature, continues to be provided to a selected group of patients, but it no longer is the theoretical treatment of choice and does not enjoy the same exceptional prestige today that it did only a decade ago.

Drug therapy, which is clearly predicated upon a medical, somatic conception of illness, is popularly credited with being instrumental in the reduction of hospital inpatient populations. Reports from New York State mental hospitals (Brill & Patton, 1959) and elsewhere regarding the efficacy of drugs with acute and chronic patients, received widespread acceptance and led to the common usage of this treatment modality. Even in institutions where almost every patient received psychotherapy at least once a week, drugs were also administered routinely (Burdock et al., 1961). More recently, May's (1968) studies of the comparative efficacy of drug, verbal and social treatment techniques led him to conclude that drugs are the most effective single treatment with the average acute schizophrenic patient. Similar findings were obtained by Grinspoon, Ewalt, & Shader (1968) in their studies with chronically schizophrenic patients. It is clear that drug therapy has assumed increasing importance and prestige within the clinical armamentarium, and this in turn often reinforces the orientation of psychiatric facilities toward dealing primarily with problems responsive to medical and physical intervention techniques.

Earlier in this chapter we noted that although nineteenth-century psychiatrists had conceived of insanity in somatic terms, they recognized that hospital treatment programs should include psychologically healthy environments as well as medication. With the demise of moral therapy, however, the milieu of the mental hospital suffered from decades of neglect, and it was not until after World War II that sustained effort was directed at reestablishing a humane institutional environment. Steps were taken to upgrade the physical and social atmosphere of wards to maximize the therapeutic potential of both patients and staff, and many dehumanizing practices were eliminated or curtailed. For example, such symbols of prison psychology as seclusion rooms and closed wards became less commonplace as it was realized that they were necessary primarily because of the breakdown in relations between staff and patients.

As the patient's right to freedom and dignity received greater attention, more emphasis was placed upon the therapeutic milieu as a clinical technique through which disturbed individuals could relearn vitally needed interpersonal skills. Stanton & Schwartz's (1954) classic study of interaction patterns within hospital milieus demonstrated that clinical technology could be considerably enhanced by integrating sociodynamic and psychodynamic concepts. The reports of Jones (1953) and Greenblatt, Levinson, & Williams (1957) further demonstrated that patients could therapeutically be assimilated into many levels of hospital life, from participating in simple decisions about daily living arrangements to collaborating with administrators about complex issues affecting basic institutional policy. An equally significant development was the fact that lower-level staff members, who had been subjected to many of the same indignities as patients, were invigorated with a sense of importance and their latent skills and creativity became powerful therapeutic forces.

The rationale of the therapeutic milieu was further elaborated by the Cummings (1962), who related ego psychology to social system theory in designing ward treatment programs. During the 1960s, the principles of the therapeutic community won numerous adherents, and these programs flourished, particularly in those facilities where the etiology of mental illness was thought to be rooted in interpersonal conflict. For example, much of the inpatient treatment program at the Fort Logan Mental Health Center was focused on therapeutic milieus, and Kraft (1963) noted that an unresolved issue was how to extend each staff member's "therapeutic self" without causing him to lose his professional identity. Based upon the therapeutic community's philosophy that patients can learn social skills, a variety of rehabilitation programs have been developed to teach patients occupational skills as well. Milieus like sheltered workshops and halfway houses have proliferated, and they try to realize the potential remaining even in chronic patients by providing meaningful rewards and incentives.

The past impact of social therapy ideas in rejuvenating dispirited, inhumane hospital settings is clearly evident. The future utility of these concepts as a clinical technology is more questionable, however. Reviews by Zeitlyn (1967) and Stotsky & Margolin (1967) have pointed up significant limitations as well as benefits in the therapeutic community, and research by May (1968) and Spadoni & Smith (1969) found this technology to be relatively ineffective in treating acute schizophrenics.

Finally, behavioral modification technologies have received growing attention and are being utilized in scores of mental hospitals because of their particular suitability to the treatment of longterm hospitalized patients. Despite London's (1972) assertion that behavioral therapy is based less on theory than on ideology, most observers agree that learning principles have been successfully refined and applied for the remediation of inappropriate behavior. A major impetus for the use of behavioral modification technologies with psychiatric inpatients stemmed from the work of Ayllon & Azrin (1968) who employed a token economy for back-ward, female chronic schizophrenics. Their finding that reinforcement contingencies can produce desired behavior among regressed individuals has been replicated in many other programs. Kazdin & Bootzin's (1972) review of the burgeoning relevant literature led them to conclude that the effectiveness of token reinforcements in increasing the frequency of a target response among hospitalized patients seems well-established. They cautioned, however, that it is also necessary to know whether the achieved gains will be maintained in settings outside the hospital. Unfortunately, the issue of response-generalization has received little empirical investigation in token reinforcement programs.

It is clear that community-oriented mental hospitals will have to continue seeking new clinical technologies if they are to deal with the wide variety of problems confronting them. The new techniques may range from hiring nonprofessionals to perform functions which previously had been limited to professionals, e.g. screening and therapy, to the involvement of professionals in tasks which formerly were considered nonprofessional in nature, e.g. stimulating social-action programs. Mental hospitals favoring the medical model of illness may be expected to retain traditional clinical technologies and to experiment particularly with new somatic ones. On the other hand, mental hospitals pursuing the interpersonal problems-in-living approach will increasingly utilize novel technologies and experiment with such modalities as sensitivity training and family therapy.

Even if increased emphasis is placed upon innovative clinical technology, this will not suffice if we do not similarly modify the administrative structures through which comprehensive clinical programs are operated. Treatment programs are not conducted in an organizational vacuum; they are profoundly affected by such administrative variables as communication patterns, leadership styles, decisionmaking processes and interorganizational relationships.

Ideally, the hospital's administrative structure should facilitate specific treatment approaches and impose minimal constraints upon the professional staff. Such is the case in at least some institutions, but many more are still burdened by historical legacies which perpetuate the need to function simultaneously as penal institution, poorhouse, general hospital and educational facility. The administrative patterns for fulfilling these different functions vary, and yet the mental hospital often is required to incorporate all of them into one structure. Thus, it is not surprising to find that a hospital's administrative structure is suitable for some of its purposes but not for others. The traditional pattern under which the superintendent and clinical director maintain tight control over patients and staff is appropriate for the hospital's custodial functions; it is antithetical, however, to its educational and rehabilitative purposes which require flexibility and spontaneity. Szasz (1961) and others have long pointed to the anomalies created for patient treatment by confused organizational patterns, and the clarification of these problems has finally assumed a new significance.

The organizational structures of community-oriented mental hospitals have evolved in a number of directions over the past two decades. Among the most widereaching administrative strategies for achieving contemporary goals is the unit plan, through which a large hospital is divided into decentralized sections, each of which provides comprehensive services to its assigned patients. The unit maintains clinical and administrative responsibility for the patient throughout his course of treatment so that continuity of care may be increased while depersonalization is reduced (Schulberg & Baker, 1969).

The changing way in which patients have been assigned to decentralized units is an excellent index of the mental hospital's evolution from its former primary focus upon in-patient care to a community orientation. Under the pioneering unit plans of the early 1950s, patients were randomly distributed among all of the inpatient sections. By the 1960s, however, it generally was proposed that each unit assume responsibility for a specific geographic area and treat all patients coming from it. With this new catchment-area focus, hospital staff can relate more easily to the community and its varied caregivers and thus participate with local agencies in the planning and operation of necessary programs.

Together with the attention now being focused upon the mental hospital's internal organization, it also is necessary to consider the possible administrative patterns whereby the hospital relates to other resources in the caregiving network. As we indicated earlier, the specific pattern which the hospital decides to pursue most often is related to its conception of community mental health ideology and programs. Auerswald (1969), for example, has described an ecological systems strategy for the prevention, diagnosis and treatment of disturbed youngsters which emphasizes the multidetermined nature of behavioral symptoms. Here, the psychiatric facility is but one part of a larger human services network which collectively provides its community with necessary biopsychosocial care. The participation of all facilities is needed to resolve individual problems and community tensions. An example of a different step in the direction of improved interorganizational relations is that of the consortium established by a group of six Philadelphia hospitals (Leopold, 1967) to insure that the totality of their integrated program would be greater than the sum of their individual services. This arrangement is more akin to the medical organizational network in that it was organized and administered by departments of psychiatry. The consortium recognized, however, that wherever necessary it must create and operate facilities and services in addition to those of the member institutions.

Professional Identities

Ideology is an important factor affecting both the development and the maintenance of an individual's role-conception within his professional work setting. Levinson (1959) has stated that "if ideology portrays and rationalizes the organizational world, then role-conception delineates the specific functioning appropriate to one's position within it [p. 276]." The psychological functions of an ideology for the individual were described by Sharaf & Levinson (1959) in their analysis of the manner in which psychiatric residents select role-definitions. In a mental hospital which reflects competing ideologies about the organization of psychiatric services, the choice of a specific orientation serves to reduce the professional's anxiety and to define his specific functions.

As ideological perspectives change, role-definitions change as well. Colleagues develop different expectations of the role-incumbent, and conflict will result unless he is in concert with the modified expectations. Community mental health ideology, with its greater emphasis upon getting a job done than upon the discipline of the person who performs it, is particularly capable of upsetting professional identities and blurring career lines. In a review of factors affecting interprofessional relations and the utilization of personnel in community mental health programs, Schulberg & Baker (1970) have reported the following trends which may well affect personnel-utilization in the changing mental hospital.

1. The composition of mental health teams is changing as programs become more sensitive to social concerns and the effects of poverty, racism and the complexities of urban life. These personnel changes are particularly evident within those mental hospitals participating in a human services network. Indigenous nonprofessionals are being recruited to perform a variety of tasks of both a clinical and nonclinical nature because of their easier access to and rapport with the local community. As a result, some groups of professionals will experience shifts in their levels of influence and prestige. In the past, psychiatrists operating within a medical model of

illness have been particularly concerned about sharing tasks with groups considered incapable of performing them, and it is these professionals who are exhibiting the greatest concern about the changing composition of mental health teams.

2. The nature of the generalist and specialist functions of each team member remain to be clarified. Even though these functions are in many ways antithetical, the aim of many training programs is to: (a) develop personnel who share an essential core-education, and (b) provide them with the skills unique to their particular discipline. Within the intrapsychically oriented mental hospital, psychotherapy, for example, has generally been a shared service provided by psychiatrists, psychologists and social workers even though each discipline still retained its unique responsibilities. A problems-in-living approach will require a reanalysis of the mental hospital's range of appropriate services to determine which are generalist in nature and which require the skills peculiar to a specific discipline. After several years of experimenting with the tasks performed by each discipline, Schiff (1969) concluded that the Fort Logan Mental Health Center "should have set up a process of role expansion rather than role-blurring; under role expansion, staff members would not perceive all staff members equal in performance and function, but would be given opportunities to develop and execute certain functions to the greatest degree consonant with the needs of the coordinated treatment effort [p. 264]."

3. There is growing acceptance of the viewpoint that leadership should be based upon individual competence rather than upon membership in a particular discipline. NIMH director Stanley Yolles (1966) noted that nowhere in the federal regulations about community mental health centers is it suggested that administrative leadership be limited to psychiatrists, and a growing number

of states have passed legislation which broadens the group of disciplines from which hospital and clinic administrators may be appointed. Thus, social workers and psychologists are now filling positions previously unavailable to them, particularly in programs based upon the problems-in-living model. The principle of individual competence rather than professional prerogative remains a point of contention, however, among programs organized according to a medical model. Even the well-trained nonmedical administrator who is willing to relinquish the aspiration of being director is still forced to seek the medical director's recognition as a valued colleague (Sheffel, 1967).

At any given point in time, mental hospitals are staffed by personnel at different stages of their careers. The greater the proportion of staff who have attained the "well-established" stage, the more resistant the hospital will be to ideological changes. Well-established personnel generally perceive themselves as having more to lose than gain by an ideological redefinition of their role, and the community mental health belief system will thus be treated as a threat to well-developed roles and functions. It is no surprise then to find that community mental health ideology is being received more enthusiastically by younger professionals whose career lines are still fluid than by older professionals whose professional identity is more firmly fixed.

SUMMARY

Mental health program developments during the 1950s and 1960s established a potentially viable role for the mental hospital within the framework of a comprehensive network of services. The challenge of assuming new functions and organizational structures is being met by those mental hospitals which are adopting a treatment rather than custodial orientation and are, thereby, reducing their hard-core populations. By expanding treatment programs and becoming increasingly oriented to community needs, mental hospitals are further demonstrating their relevance to the era of community mental health. The medical model of illness and the problems-in-living framework, which underlie community mental health concepts, were explored. Their implications were described for the manner in which a mental hospital defines its community, participates in a caregiving network, modifies clinical and administrative technology and utilizes professional and nonprofessional personnel.

3. *Community Mental Health Ideology*

In the absence of well-tested empirically supported models of the etiology of mental illness, mental health practitioners have tended to function largely on the basis of their beliefs about the relationships of pathological forces and illness processes in the person. As a consequence of the dynamic, changing relationship between the mental health field and the social context within which it is embedded, this relationship has been constantly reinterpreted by a succession of ideological movements which have buffeted the mental health field during the nineteenth and twentieth centuries. Each movement has produced its own unique constellation of theory and technology before falling into disrepute as the spirit of the times and the society's social, political and economic characteristics changed and weakened its support among professional adherents. From a historical perspective, perhaps the most striking aspect of this phenomenon is the fact that as mental health professionals continue to pass through cycles of social and cultural revolution they find that it is just as productive to resurrect and refine mental health belief systems which had been previously discarded in disrepute as it is to create new ones.

In the 1960s the development of mental health theory and practice entered a new phase which was both hailed as "the third psychiatric revolution" (Bellak, 1964) and criticized as the "newest therapeutic band wagon" (Dunham, 1965). The accelerated pace of community mental health program development during the 1960s certainly owes much of its impetus to such recent technological developments as the widespread use of drug therapy, but most of the conceptual foundations for this ideology had already been proposed many decades earlier. A fundamental aspect of the community mental health movement is the dual emphasis of its unifying ideology upon traditional humanistic values as well as upon the modification of services so that they can meet the patient's needs. Before proceeding further, we will clarify what we mean by ideology.

The Nature of Belief-Systems

Ideology may be defined as a commonly adhered-to system of ideas or beliefs which serves to justify the position of a group and as a rationale for its behavior. By ascribing systemic qualities to the concept of ideology, emphasis is placed upon the assumption that there is a set of interrelated beliefs which may or may not be organized in a logical manner (Rokeach, 1960). The concept of a belief-system as a basis for self-definition and as a guide to behavior can be useful for understanding social groups, complex organizations and the individual. Thus, social scientists have studied belief systems concerning nations, communities, professional groups, education, religion, politics, etc. Ideology is of particular importance to the dynamic collectivity usually identified as a "social movement." Even though ideological differences have characterized the mental health field for many years, it is still painful for many professionals to have themselves collectively referred to as "movements" and to recognize the degree to which their actions reflect competing ideological commitments.

The ideological component of a social movement typically consists of four elements (Killian, 1964), and we shall examine each of these as they apply to community mental health as a new social movement. The first element is an interpretation of history which shows that the goals of the collectivity are in harmony with the traditions of the society. Bockoven (1966) described such a consonance in his analysis of the congruence in values between the American mental health establishment and American political democracy during the early and mid-1960s; the emergence of community psychiatry was characterized as paralleling the development of a new moral mandate for this country.

The second and third elements of a movement's ideology are the contrasting visions which it holds of the future—a portrayal of the frightful conditions that will prevail if the movement is not successful and a utopian vision depicting the good world which can result from the successful attainment of the collectivity's goals. The relevance of these elements to the community mental health belief-system is readily apparent in President Kennedy's message to Congress in 1963. The President called for a "bold new approach" in the treatment of mental illness and mental retardation so that the "reliance on the cold mercy of custodial isolation will be supplanted by the open warmth of community concern and capability . . . all but a small proportion of the mentally ill can eventually receive a wholesome and constructive social adjustment."

The fourth part of an ideology consists of stereotypes of the movement's heroes and villains. The type of practitioner "whose total commitment was to the private practice of psychotherapy in plush downtown offices with financially secure individuals suffering mainly from boredom or the stresses and strains of frantic pleasure-seeking" has been described by Greenblatt (1966) as a "cream puff psychiatrist." By contrast, he proudly points to his image of the new breed of community psychiatrist who is struggling to make larger contributions to society. Instead of working only with individual patients, the community psychiatrist is concerned with larger populations who are less favored in the social and occupational worlds.

A belief-system has important personality correlates as well. It attempts to understand the motivational structure of the social movement's members and their personal needs and roles in professional social systems. Levinson (1964) has formulated a "postulate of receptivity" which contends that the individual will be most receptive to those ideologies that have the greatest functional value in meeting the requirements of personality as a system. Whittington (1969) has suggested that community mental health programs, as opposed to traditional state hospital programs, tend to attract persons who are "rebellious, resentful of authority, and determined to go their own way. The result is a group likely to bring about innovation and new professional developments, but one that raises serious problems for statewide supervision and control [p. 133]."

It is important to stress that the capacity of an ideology to mobilize support depends not only on its psychological attractiveness, but also on its perceived relationship to performance. If support is to be sustained, it is necessary that members of the movement perceive that the ideology's implicit or explicit goals are being met to at least some minimal degree. If the goals that are embodied in the belief-structure fail to be achieved, in time continuing support and the attraction of new converts will begin to wane. This point both explains the decline of the earlier psychiatric ideologies which failed to deliver on their promises, and highlights the necessity for community mental health ideology to meet the expectations which it has inspired lest it suffer the same demise as its ideological predecessors. Thus, an ideology depends for its continued support on both its expressive dimensions, i.e., its capacity to enable adherents to express their personality needs, and on its instrumental capacity, i.e., its effectiveness to move men into successful action.

The Ideology of Community Mental Health

Disillusionment with ideologies emphasizing person-changing interventions designed to eliminate, or at least minimize, the consequences of mental illness, took root in the late 1950s. Sociological research in this decade demonstrated that institutionalized care not only did little to help the mentally ill but actually produced iatrogenic effects which further damaged the patient (Caudill, 1958; Goffman, 1962; Stanton & Schwartz, 1954). Humanistic concerns began to reemerge in the late 1950s and, in an attempt to lessen the harmful effects of the "total institution" (Goffman, 1962), efforts were made to transform the mental hospital from a rigid institution of incarceration to a therapeutically healthy person-oriented community. A shift from scapegoating the patient to fresh consideration of institutional social arrangements began to occur during this period.

In reviewing the ideological components of the community mental health movement, it becomes clear that widespread acceptance of this new belief system by the mental health establishment occurred as the result of professional developments as well as shifts in the greater social and political scene. The way mental illness or health is viewed in the face of changing social climates bears particular examination. Bockoven (1966) observed that the more thorough the scrutiny of the principles on which the American psychiatric and political systems are built, the more evident it becomes that they are the same ones. From this perspective, Bockoven contends that a major part of the American mental health establishment may be viewed as an arm of the humanitarian American state, and the condition designated as "mental illness" is not primarily a medical concern. Rather, mental illness is a matter of alienation and demoralization; and it is the state's responsibility to provide sanctuary and relief to those of its citizens who find themselves alienated from family and community.

Ryan (1972) has identified an analytic dimension of "exceptionalism-universalism" which is applicable to the analysis of professional beliefs about the causes and cures of mental illness. At the exceptionalist end of the continuum, the troubled individual is identified as the object of concern because of his deviation from some norm of health. Abnormality is regarded as a disease which is located inside or as a part of the person. Since the individual is viewed as the locus of the problem and even somehow at fault for having created his miserable condition, Ryan called this orientation "blaming the victim." A contrasting approach to the analysis and solution of an individual's malaise is identified by Ryan as the universalistic viewpoint whereby problems are deemed to be inclusive rather than exclusive, public rather than private, and general rather than special. According to the universalistic viewpoint, the environment and particularly the social environment is seen as the major locus of an individual's problems.

Applying Ryan's conceptual distinctions to the community mental health movement, it becomes evident that a central characteristic of this new thrust is its shift from the exceptionalist point of view toward a universalistic perspective—from a focus on the individual to a focus on large populations and their environmental situations. Hersch (1972), building on the work of Ryan (1972) and Levine & Levine (1970), has posited that individual or intrapsychic definitions of problems and helping techniques flourish in times of social-political conservatism, while situational or environmental problem definitions and modes of help tend to flourish in times of social-political reform. Therefore, it is not accidental that community mental health programs which emphasize situational modes of help and focus not only on the casualties of damaging environments but on the harmful environments themselves reached fruition during the reform-minded decade of the 1960s.

EMPIRICAL STUDIES OF IDEOLOGY

A series of empirical studies examining the ideological positions current in psychiatry during the 1950s was conducted by Levinson and his associates at the Boston Psychopathic Hospital. Gilbert & Levinson (1957) studied the distribution of ideologies among mental hospital units, using the Custodial Mental Illness (CMI) Scale, which they developed to measure custodialism and humanism as ideological orientations. They found that hospital units with the most custodial management policy were staffed by individuals with the most custodial ideologies and the most authoritarian personalities.

In a related study of two patterns of the "humanistic" orientation, Sharaf & Levinson (1957) examined the distribution of psychotherapeutic versus sociotherapeutic ideology among psychiatric residents and senior medical staff at the Boston Psychopathic Mental Hospital. Sharaf & Levinson viewed the psychotherapeutic and sociotherapeutic ideology patterns as opposite poles of the same continuum.

In a study of the orientations of practitioners providing psychiatric services to New Haven residents, Hollingshead & Redlich (1958) distinguished two other major types of therapeutic ideologies: the directiveorganic versus the analytic-psychotherapeutic. The attempt to clarify the ideological orientations of mental health workers was advanced by Strauss et al. (1964) when they integrated the somatic dimension refined by Hollingshead and Redlich with the psychotherapeutic and sociotherapeutic dimensions identified by Sharaf & Levinson. Although Strauss et al. hypothesized that each of these orientations represented a separate and distinct ideology, their data indicated that only the sociotherapeutic dimension was an independent one. The somatotherapeutic and psychotherapeutic orientations were strongly negatively correlated, suggesting the existence of a continuum of "psycho" versus "somato" ideology. Using data from a nationwide survey of hospital psychiatrists, Armor & Klerman (1968) found factor-analytic support for the independent ideologies of somatotherapy and psychotherapy. Since only a small amount of the variance could be explained by each factor, these researchers saw the need to refine their instruments and predicted that sociotherapy might develop into full ideological status under the aegis of community psychiatry.

The Community Mental Health Ideology Scale

Postulating that in the 1960s a growing collectivity of mental health professionals were forming a new social movement and beginning to share a fresh set of beliefs, the authors sought to operationally measure community mental health ideology (Baker & Schulberg, 1967). In reviewing the literature to construct an objective scale of personal commitment to community mental health, we found that the common beliefs of its exponents could be conceptually categorized into the following five themes:

1. *A population focus.* The view that the mental health specialist should be responsible not only for individual patients with whom he has contracted for treatment, but for the entire population of both identified and unidentified potentially sick members in his community.

2. *Primary prevention.* The concept of lowering the rate of new cases of mental disorder in a population by counteracting harmful forces before they have had a chance to produce illness.

3. *Social treatment goals.* The belief that the primary goal of treatment is not to reconstruct the mental patient's personality, but rather to help him achieve social adjustment in an ordinary life situation as soon as possible.

4. *Comprehensive continuity of care.* The view that there should be a continuity of professional responsibility as the patient moves from one program to another in an integrated network of caregiving services.

5. *Total community involvement.* The belief that the mental health specialist is only one member of a group of community agents caring for the mentally ill and that he can extend his effectiveness by work with and through other people.

Eighty-eight declarative statements, worded both positively and negatively, were constructed on the basis of these five conceptual categories so as to insure that major aspects of the community mental health ideology were covered. In order to refine the scale's content validity, the 88-item preliminary questionnaire was submitted to a nationwide panel of 16 judges composed of nationally known individuals from different disciplines who had been prominently identified with the community mental health movement through either their writings or their clinical programs. These judges were asked to rate the degree to which an "agree" and "disagree" response to each item would reflect a respondent's endorsement of a community mental health orientation. On the basis of a sufficient consensus among the judges, and considerations of a distribution of item-extremity to give a sufficiently wide and representative span to the full gamut of opinion, items were selected from the initial pool and some items were rewritten in accord with the judges' suggestions. The 64 items resulting from this initial assessment of content validity were arranged in a Likert response-format questionnaire and distributed for completion to a nationwide sample of 484 mental health specialists from nine criterion groups. The respondents were sampled from four criterion groups whose members were thought to be highly oriented to community mental health, three national professional associations and two professional groups which it was assumed would include psychiatrists more negatively oriented toward community mental health ideology.

The final version of the instrument labeled the Community Mental Health Ideology (CMHI) Scale is composed of items selected on the basis of item-total correlations and the results of a principal-components analysis of the 64-item questionnaire. Thirty-eight items were found to have corrected item-total correlations of .44 or higher and factor loadings of .44 or higher on the first factor of the principal-components analysis. These 38 items (19 positively and 19 negatively worded) comprise the refined form of the CMHI Scale.

The CMHI Scale is arranged in Likert-type attitude scale format, with provision being made for respondents to circle one of six response categories for each item: strongly, moderately, or slightly agree; and strongly, moderately, or slightly disagree. On positively worded items, strong agreement is scored seven and strong disagreement one, with intermediate scores given to other levels of agreement and disagreement. Reverse scoring is used for negatively worded items. When no clear response is given, a score of four is assigned to that item. Some examples of the CMHI Scale* items are:

> —A mental health program should direct particular attention to groups of people who are potentially vulnerable to upsetting pressures.
> —The mental health specialist should seek to extend his effectiveness by working through other people.
> —The locus of mental illness must be viewed as extending beyond the individual, and into the family, the community, and society.
> —The responsible mental health professional should become an agent for social change.

The initial evidence indicates that reliability for the CMHI Scale is quite acceptable. The Cronbach Alpha (generalized Kuder-Richardson formula 20) for the group of respondents on which the scale was originally developed is .94, and a split-half reliability of .92 was obtained (Baker and Schulberg, 1967).

Initial evidence for the validity of the CMHI Scale included research findings indicating that the scale successfully discriminated groups known to have positive community mental health views from random samples of mental health professionals. CMHI Scale scores were also shown to relate significantly to self-reported questionnaire responses on degree of: identification with a

*The Community Mental Health Ideology Scale is published by Behavioral Publications, 72 Fifth Avenue, New York, N.Y. 10011, and is available in printed form with scoring keys and a manual from the publisher.

community mental health orientation, interest in keeping up with new developments in community mental health and preference for a symposium on recent advances in community mental health (Baker & Schulberg, 1967). Scores on the CMHI Scale were also shown to relate significantly to the connotative meanings assigned community mental health on a 19-item semantic differential rating form (Schulberg & Baker, 1967).

Subsequent research has provided additional evidence of the reliability and validity of the CMHI Scale. Langston (1970) administered the CMHI Scale to all employees of two community mental health centers in Houston, Texas. His data essentially replicated Baker & Schulberg's initial study of the scale's validity by successfully discriminating samples of some of the same professional criterion groups examined in the basic research. Breeskin et al. (1972) employed the CMHI Scale in a survey of all active-duty United States Air Force clinical psychologists, psychiatrists and psychiatric social workers as of 1970–1971. They also surveyed an additional sample of mental health professionals working, on a voluntary basis, at the Washington Free Clinic in Washington, D.C., a group described by Breeskin and his colleagues as comprised of "individuals who are actively engaged in innovative mental health settings [p. 5]." Breeskin et al. found that the CMHI Scale clearly differentiated among professional groups in the Air Force, and that the Air Force mental health professionals had a significantly lower average Community Mental Health Ideology Scale score than the mental health professionals drawn from the same disciplines working in the Free Clinic.

Two further studies have obtained results which support the validity of the Community Mental Health Ideology Scale with regard to the criteria of professional role-definition and choice of work situation. In a nationwide survey of graduate students in psychiatric nursing, Howard & Baker (1971) asked 368 graduate student nurses to complete the Community Mental Health Ideology Scale and also to evaluate a list of 22 role-activities for their importance as functions within the nurse's community mental health role. Nurses with high scores on the CMHI Scale, as compared to nurses with lower scores, tended to emphasize a wider range of community-oriented activities as appropriate. Gross (1972) compared individuals with high and low CMHI Scale scores in terms of whether or not they chose to work in a community setting. He found that mental health workers with a strong commitment to community mental health ideology were more likely to make the behavioral choice of working in a community setting than those with low commitment to this orientation.

Correlates of Community Mental Health Ideology

The relationship of community mental health ideology to other characteristics of mental health professionals has been studied in a number of ways. Baker & Schulberg (1967) found that respondents with high scores on the CMHI Scale differed from low scorers in terms of how they spent their work week and in the type of work setting in which they were employed. Respondents in the highest-scoring quartile on total CMHI Scale scores spent a significantly greater proportion of their time in administration, consulting with community agencies and teaching than did respondents in the lowest-scoring quartile. The members of the high group spent an average of over 50% of their time in these activities as compared to those in the lowest group, who devoted only a quarter of their work week to these three types of activities. In contrast, the lowest-scoring group spent significantly more of its work week in treating patients than did respondents with CMHI scores placing them in the highest quartile. Baker & Schulberg also found that a greater proportion of community mental health–oriented professionals work in universities and medical schools, general hospitals, community clinics and school systems than do less community mental health–oriented individuals, of whom a greater proportion worked in mental hospitals. Additionally, three times as many of the lowest-scoring group spent the majority of their professional work week in private practice as compared to the highest-scoring group.

The relationship between age and community mental health orientation has been found to be significantly correlated (Baker & Schulberg, 1967); those supporting community mental health beliefs tend to be younger. There is a similarly significant correlation between a high total score and recency of highest educational degree, indicating that individuals receiving advanced training in the past several years are more likely to have been socialized to a community mental health orientation.

Support of an ideology depends on "its capacity to enable adherents to express their personality needs [Baker & Schulberg, 1969, pp. 16–17]." Penn, Baker, & Schulberg (1973) studied the relationship of personality characteristics and community mental health ideology among graduate students in social work. They administered the CMHI Scale and the Edwards Personal Preference Schedule (EPPS) to 105 women graduate students enrolled in four schools of social work in the Greater Boston area. Results of this study indicated that the degree of commitment to community mental health ideology is significantly related to two of the personality preferences measured by the EPPS: needs for order and deference. Social work students who showed a strong orientation to the community mental health belief system, when compared to those showing a low degree of belief, had significantly less needs for deference and order.

The relationship between community mental health ideology and other personality and idea systems has also been explored by Baker & Schulberg (1969). Since community mental health ideology includes many nontraditional beliefs aimed at greater social involvement with persons experiencing difficulty in adjusting to their environment, it was thought particularly relevant to measure the relationship of this ideology to the variables of dogmatism, and liberalism versus conservatism. Rokeach (1960) and Vacchiano et al. (1968) contend that dogmatism is a general personality trait related to one's ability to form new conceptual systems, while the dimension of liberalism versus conservatism was found to be integral to the assessment of the authoritarian personality (Adorno et al., 1950). Baker & Schulberg administered the CMHI Scale, an abridged version of Rokeach's Dogmatism Scale and the five-item form of the Political-Economic-Conservatism Scale to 140 members of the Massachusetts Citizen Mental Health Area Boards. The results indicated that degree of adherence to community mental health ideology as measured by the CMHI Scale is significantly negatively correlated with dogmatism and political-economic conservatism. Baker and Schulberg found that the sample of nonprofessional citizens scored higher on the CMHI Scale than had groups of previously studied mental health professionals, suggesting that the impetus for planning innovative community-oriented services might better stem from citizens than professionals.

SUMMARY

During the 1960s, mental health professionals expanded the scope of their activities and perspectives from the relatively insular mental hospital and clinic to the more inclusive community mental health program. This development coincided with and is related to the emergence of a new belief system, community mental health ideology, as a dominant mental health theory and practice. Empirical research with the Community Mental Health Ideology Scale demonstrated that this new ideological orientation exists as a major belief system among a variety of professional groups and that the degree of commitment to this new approach varies across and among professional disciplines. Research also showed that commitment to this new orientation is associated with work setting, recency of training, low needs for order and deference, nondogmatism and liberalism.

As mental hospitals are reevaluated with regard to their role in the community and challenged by new organizational arrangements such as the community mental health center, staff's acceptance or resistance to emerging psychiatric ideologies is an important factor affecting capacity for program change and development. Thus, analysis of the intensity of ideological patterns and their distribution among hospital staff is vital for understanding the widely differing acceptance and development of community-oriented services within traditional mental health organizations.

4. *An Open Systems Approach to Mental Health Program Development*

A major problem in developing a comprehensive community mental health network is that of conceptualizing the organization and operation of any single component program, such as a mental hospital, in relation to the other relevant community caregiving resources. The authors have attempted to grapple with this problem by refining an open systems approach which is useful for conceptualizing the organizational issues in mental health program development (Baker, 1969a; Schulberg, Sheldon, & Baker, 1969; Baker, 1970; Baker & Schulberg, 1970; Schulberg & Baker, 1970; Baker, 1971; Baker & O'Brien, 1971; Baker, 1972; Baker & Schulberg, 1973; Baker, 1973a, 1973b). The major goal of this chapter is to present an integrated overview and application of general systems concepts to the examination of the mental hospital as an open organizational system operating in a complex interorganizational field of human services providers.

OPEN SYSTEMS

The growth of a literature conceptualizing organizations as open systems has taken place largely within the last decade. Much of the stimulus for this point of view has come from the development of general systems theory in biology with its emphasis on systems interdependencies and the importance of openness to the environment as a characteristic of all living systems, including such large social systems as complex organizations.

Systems approaches, theory and research currently nave very widespread popularity. A major clustering in the systems movement consists of those individuals from a variety of widely different disciplines who are striving for a "general systems theory," a body of organized theoretical constructs which can be employed to discuss the general relationships of empirical phenomena ranging from biological systems to social systems. Ludwig von Bertalanffy, a theoretical biologist, is generally credited with founding the general systems movement. In a now-classic paper, Bertalanffy (1950) elaborated a rigorous distinction between living and nonliving systems on the basis of their "openness" to the environment. Bertalanffy asserted that all living or open systems differ from nonliving or closed systems in that open systems require a continuous flow of resources from the environment and a continuous outflow of products of the systems action back to the environment. Viewing human organizations as open systems stresses the dependence of such enterprises for growth and viability upon their processes and transactions with environment.

A system is essentially defined as a set of units or elements which are actively interrelated and operate in some sense as a bounded unit (Baker, 1969b; Bertalanffy, 1956; Hall & Fagen, 1956; Ackoff, 1960; Miller, 1965a). Miller has noted that organizations exist at one level in a hierarchy of living systems which is characterized by isomorphic properties which permit generalization about the behavior of systems across levels, including the individual, the group and the organization among others (Miller, 1965a). The pattern of activities of an open system is characterized by an active matter-energy and information exchange with an external environment across a boundary, which possesses the property of determining the flow of inputs and outputs into and out of the system. The inputs admitted to a system are transformed or reorganized through the application of *throughput* processes. For example, an organization creates a new product, processes materials, trains people or provides a service. In turn, some of this modified input is exported to the environment as output and becomes available for use as inputs for other systems. A portion of the output may be returned as input to the system so as to modify succeeding outputs of the system, a process known as *feedback*.

Miller (1965a) viewed a living system as self-regulating since not only does input affect output, but output often adjusts input. *Negative feedback* describes a situation in which information comes back to the system as input in such a way as to decrease the deviation of output from a steady state. *Positive feedback* occurs when information comes back to a system over a feedback channel in such a way that these signals increase the deviation of the output from some previous level.

It is possible to identify smaller units or components which singly or in combination with other system units play specialized roles in the operation of the larger system. These subsystems can be analyzed in terms of their structure and processes. As Miller (1965b) explains, relationships among subsystems or components involve either structures or processes; the structural relationships are spatial in character and the process relationships are either purely temporal or involve spatial changes in time. In an open system, at least three types of subsystems can be identified which are associated with the three major aspects of the system's cyclic character: an input subsystem functioning to accept inputs; a conversion subsystem functioning to modify inputs; and an output subsystem functioning to export new products

FIGURE 4-1
Operating Process Flow of a Simple Formal Organizational System*

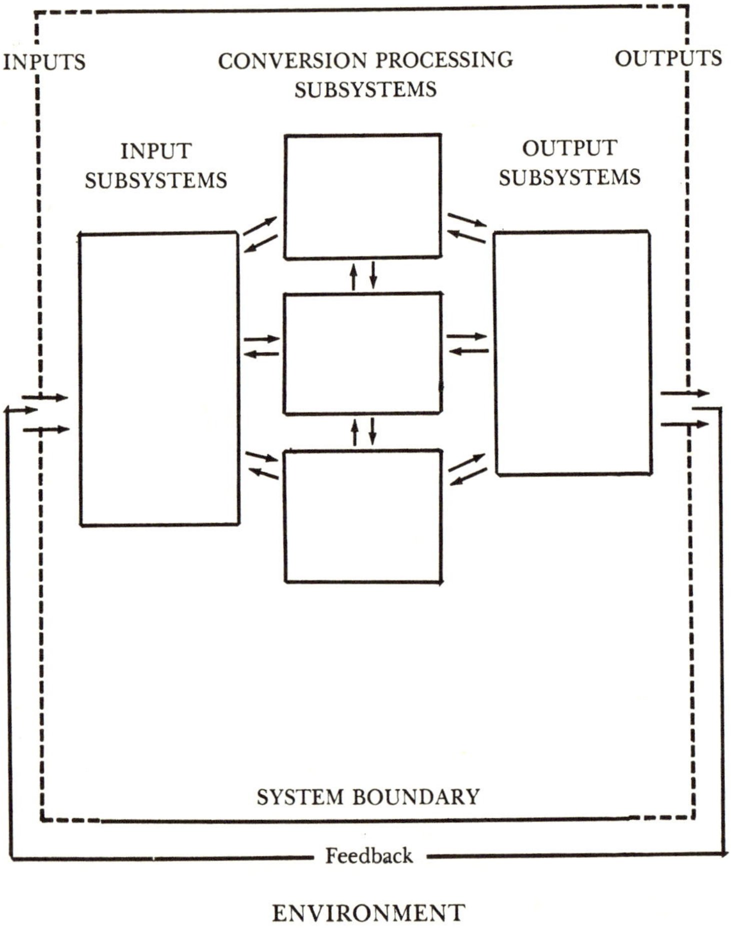

*This is a simplified and highly stylized diagram of the input-throughput-output-feedback flow through a formal organizational system. It is not intended to represent the full complexity of most organizations, and for the sake of simplicity does not show managerial subsystems of informal communication structures.

Although shown as a single line, the feedback loop represents numerous feedback channels. Internal feedback is represented by reversed arrows (⇄).

of the system's throughput activities. The operating flow of a simple organizational system is schematically represented in Figure 4-1.

Sociotechnical Systems Model

Perhaps the most extensive body of theoretical and empirical work applying the systems perspective at the level of internal organizational processes is the sociotechnical systems theory developed over the past two decades by such behavioral scientists as Trist, Emery, Rice and Eric Miller at London's Tavistock Institute of Human Relations. Originally influenced by Bertalanffy's delineation of open systems, the concept of a sociotechnical system was developed from analyses of production systems (Trist & Bamforth, 1951). It was recognized that such systems require technological components (e.g., machinery, raw materials and plant layout) as well as social components which structure the work relationship relating the human operators both to the technology and to each other (Emery & Trist, 1960).

Human relationists and behavioral scientists have focused on the psychosocial subsystem, and management scientists have emphasized technical and economic subsystems. The sociotechnical system model emphasizes that in a systemic approach to work organizations, both the technological and the social components of a productive organization must be considered, since technology and social systems mutually influence one another.

The Open People-Belief-Resource Systems Model

Open systems models like the sociotechnical systems model hold much promise for useful application to mental health and related human resource organizations, but there have been relatively few studies of such organizations based on these conceptual models. Perhaps this gap is attributable to the lack of appropriate adaptations of open systems concepts to mental health and other human services organizations. In this chapter, we consequently are concerned with outlining the elements of an open systems model of human services organizations which integrates several concepts previously employed by general system thinkers.

People are a basic component of any organizational system. The Tavistock group emphasized this in their concept of the sociotechnical system; "socio" highlights the sociopsychological or the people-dimension of the system (Trist et al., 1963). In the industrial production organizations of primary concern to the Tavistock group, the people intimately involved in the organization's functioning are basically the individuals employed by the organization. The distinction between consumer and organizational member, however, is less distinct in the human services organization (HSO). This was emphasized by the research of the 1950s which examined such custodial institutions as the mental hospital, and stressed the importance of patients, or clients, as an important part of the treatment organization as well as the professional staff who worked in that type of HSO (Caudill, 1958; Goffman, 1961; Stanton & Schwartz, 1954). People are not only important components of the HSO system in setting goals and determining outputs, but they are important because they are also that which is processed by this type of system. In an industrial production organization, the customers are external to the system, while in an HSO the clients may be considered to be part of the human components which comprise the system. Thus, through interactive effects with the staff of the HSO the client will not only be changed by the system" pertains to the degree to which the technological

The "technical" part of the concept "sociotechnical system," pertains to the degree to which the technological demands of industrial production organizations determine structures and processes. While technology is certainly important in the human services organization, many types of HSO's lack a clear base of demonstrably effective technology. This is perhaps particularly true with mental health and social service organizations as was suggested in Chapters 2 and 3. They consequently depend more on the attitudes, values, beliefs and ideologies of the professional staff concerning the ideal patterns of conduct and ideal goal states.

A number of studies have shown the importance of belief-systems for the professionals who work in human services organizations. Wessen (1958) demonstrated that a general hospital is characterized by a set of disparate institutional ideologies which limit the degree to which various professional work groups can be integrated. In Chapter 3 we reviewed the work of Levinson and his associates (Gilbert & Levinson, 1957; Sharaf & Levinson, 1957), who found that psychiatric ideological positions of the 1950s related to the degree of custodial care offered in the mental hospital, and the work of Strauss et al. (1964), who studied the psychotherapeutic, somatotherapeutic and sociotherapeutic orientations. As they concluded after their study of several psychiatric institutions, "Ideology makes a difference in the organization of treatment: in what is done to and for patients and in the accompanying division of labor [p. 361]."

Community mental health ideology has similar broad implications for the pattern of services offered in contemporary mental health organizations. Thus, professional beliefs undoubtedly play a significant role in human services organizational systems by determining the types of service offered and the manner in which patients or clients are treated.

Until recently, the beliefs and values of professionals have tended to prevail over consumer values in the structuring and functioning of HSOs. Although in some sense mental health and social welfare organizations have always been responsible to the public interest and the needs of a larger community, they have lacked the direct feedback linkages available to profitmaking organizations in the latter's economic relationships to the marketplace. Although human services organizations are increasingly accountable to their actual or potential clients, there is still a strong tendency for the goals and performance criteria of HSO's to be determined on the basis of professional rather than consumer criteria and value judgments.

In addition to people and their beliefs, another major category of elements integral to a human services organization is that of its nonhuman resources such as buildings, equipments, materials and financial assets. Gross (1966) has pointed out that nonhuman resources do not exist apart from people. He observes that "physical objects can become resources only when two conditions are met: (1) when there are people with certain interests to be satisfied, and (2) when there are people with the knowledge and technological know-how required to use such physical objects to the satisfaction of such interests [Gross, 1966, p. 192]." While the people-processing HSO lacks the well-developed machine technology associated with the production of commercial products in an industrial organization, nonhuman resources do play a significant role in this type of organizational system, particularly as they relate to professional values.

A human services organization thus may be conceptualized as an open *people-belief-resource* (PBR) *system*. The HSO is a living system expressive of the prevailing beliefs, ideology and values which guide the actions of the people comprising this system, as well as indicative of the way they utilize various nonhuman resources. The major dimensions of the human services organization are defined by the beliefs and capacities of its people in interaction with available nonhuman resources, both being influenced by environmental conditions.

Causal Texture of the Environment

A major problem in planning and managing organizational change is that the environmental contexts in which most contemporary organizations exist are themselves undergoing change at an increasing rate in the direction of growing complexity. Mental hospitals moving toward a community orientation, along with other human services organizations, can be conceptualized as operating under a variety of differing environmental conditions. Emery & Trist (1965) have referred to these conditions as differences in the causal texture, and they have performed an important service by classifying a number of environmental types. Emery & Trist conceptualize a continuum on which causal texture differs in the degree of uncertainty and in the degree of interdependence exhibited among the parts or regions of the environment. According to this continuum, society can be seen as moving from a time in which conditions were relatively placid and certain to an era in which organizations must operate in "turbulent" circumstances. The turbulence results not simply from the increased interaction of identifiable component systems, but from the complexity and multiple character of the causal interconnections of the environmental field itself.

It is becoming increasingly apparent that, like other human services organizations, community-oriented mental hospitals must operate in environments characterized by turbulence. The environmental turbulence is being increased by the expansion of science and technology, by changes in societal values, by changes in professions and notably by the growing aspirations of people throughout the society to control rather than to be victims of their surroundings.

FOUR GENERAL SYSTEMS FUNCTIONS

In order to survive and maintain some degree of autonomy of action in a "turbulent" environment, a mental hospital like other human services organizations must fulfill a number of important functions. It must deal with the external environment in such a way that it can acquire and maintain sufficient levels of necessary resources, as well as adapt to the environment itself. Thus, at times the mental hospital as a total system will take a reactive stance with regard to the environment, responding to task demands generated from without. At other times the organization will take a proactive stance in response to internally generated demands for more resources and will initiate activity which attempts to modify environmental conditions so as to improve the organization's overall position with regard to resource-acquisition.

Four general systems functions may be identified which an organizational system must fulfill in order to maintain autonomy and insure continued survival. It must (1) acquire inputs and deliver outputs, (2) develop system goals, (3) achieve integration and coordination subsystems in the face of differentiating environmental influence, and (4) adapt to both the environment and its internal requirements, and to some degree try to control or adapt the environment itself.

Our open systems conceptual framework for analyzing mental hospital program development grows out of an elaboration and consideration of each of these four key functions of any organizational system.

Acquisition of Inputs and Delivery of Outputs

Environmental characteristics and resource availability define the nature of inputs. An organizational system's input variables in turn define the character of a total organizational system as they are operated upon at various times and in multiple ways. Organizational inputs both determine and are modified by subsystems, structures and processes. As a result of the internal processing of inputs, output variables are produced, and it is these alone that are usually considered in defining the system's effectiveness. Basic to the conception of an organization as an open system is the assumption that any enterprise, or parts of it, can be characterized as admitting inputs from the environment, converting or transforming them and delivering outputs back to the environment.

Inputs of numerous sorts constitute the variables which, when operated on in various ways, determine the outputs. The subsystem's variables, the internal structures, attitudes and activities account for the conversion or transformation of the inputs into outputs. These three sets of variables—input, throughput, output—constitute the very core of the open system organizational model which was employed in our study of a changing mental hospital.

A major category of input for a people-processing organization like a mental hospital is that of the individuals defined as patients. The qualitative and quantitative aspects of the raw material available from the environment to an industrial system are major constraints on its productivity. Similarly, the characteristics of patients admitted to the mental hospital may be examined in terms of demographic characteristics such as age, sex and education which abet or limit therapeutic success. History of previous illness, for example, poses a major constraint on the hospital's ability to treat its patients successfully and return them to the community. Thus, the nature of the population served by the hospital is extremely important in determining the system's functioning and effectiveness. As the mental hospital takes responsibility for a specific geographic catchment area, changes will result in the input character of patients to the system. As a consequence of these changes in the system's patient input, the internal structure and functions of the hospital and the character of its output will be similarly affected. For example, as an increasing number of individuals are treated on an outpatient basis, the balance between hospital-based and community-based programs is bound to be altered.

Another kind of human input relevant to our analysis is the personnel coming into the hospital system, including the fully trained professionals as well as the residents, student nurses and others who receive professional training in the hospital system. Human beings are not passive materials or instruments of treatment. As opposed to nonhuman materials, human input is highly reactive; the personal response dispositions and abilities of both patients and staff are important input variables which act to constrain the hospital systems operation. The level and type of professional staff skills, their personalities, attitudes, interests, goals, ideologies and habits are thus important variables to consider as they affect the organization in all of its functions.

In addition to human inputs, a hospital must also receive material inputs of money, supplies, and facilities. A mental hospital's interaction with its environmental sources of political, legal and financial support largely determines the limits of its ultimate output. Human and nonhuman resources, as they are assembled, determine and define the very nature of the total organizational system since it is the aggregation of interacting parts.

Open organizational systems must acquire resources to survive. Typically, an organization seeks to improve its survival position by stockpiling reserves to endure a comfortable margin of operation. Nevertheless, in order to maintain itself and to grow, an organization must regularly direct a major part of its activities toward resource-acquisition. Its pattern of functioning at any given time, thus, will be determined by its success in controlling the flow into the system of needed human and material resources.

Acquisition of resources is dependent, however indirectly, upon the continued production by the organization of needed goods and services. For environmental constituents, the reason for supporting an organization is its ability to deliver desirable outputs. As was mentioned above, human services organizations, like mental hospitals, have been less constrained by a "market" economy but are increasingly being held accountable within a framework of evolving criteria. Environmental constituents differ, however, in the value which they assign to such intangible products as human services. Society's values with regard to the treated mentally ill have undergone cyclical change; thus, the acceptable patient output mix of the mental hospital tends to be basically unstable over time.

DEVELOPMENT OF SYSTEM GOALS

Organizations have been distinguished from small groups on the basis of their formal character as planned structures for the achievement of specific goals. Classical organization theory restricted the study of formal organizations to the conscious, planned, rational aspects of organizations, and classical models were primarily concerned with the specification of the necessary division of labor for accomplishing specific goals. In attempting to develop a model of an organization capable of attaining goals, there has often been a tendency to give inadequate attention to relationships among roles and among other elements of the organization. It is important to distinguish a goal-attainment model from a systems model in the specific implications that each approach has for the design, management and evaluation of developing mental hospital programs. Although the systems model is often contrasted with the more traditional goal model, the systems model is neither divorced from nor in opposition to this approach. The organizational system must in fact organize its human and material resources toward articulated ends in order to achieve future outcomes. Differences between the two models, however, are important to delineate.

A goal-attainment model directs the evaluator's attention to final outcome analysis. By contrast, an open systems model of an organization leads a researcher to focus not only on final outcome analysis, but also on process-oriented analysis including examination of the intermediate outputs of the system. In the goal model, the structure and processes of an organization are treated largely as a "black box"; in other words, the insides of the organization are ignored and the organization is viewed predominantly in terms of an anticipated output.

There are several serious weaknesses to the goal model. One of the principal problems is that this model overemphasizes goal-achievement as a determining factor of organizational effectiveness and success. Obviously in determining whether goals are being maximized, one needs some surety in the establishment of the goals that are to be assessed. Frequently, however, discrepancies arise between stated goals which receive the majority of the organization's resources and the major commitments of the organizational membership. The goals stated by organizational spokesmen, or the goals contained in charters or other documents, are likely to be mainly for public consumption. As Etzioni (1960) has pointed out, the goals which an organization claims to pursue "fail to be realized . . . because . . . they are not meant to be realized [p. 260]." If an organizational analyst evaluates a complex organization solely in terms of goals, omitting consideration of other aspects of a system, he is likely to find himself devoting a good part of his study's written report to describing the focal organization's lack of goal-accomplishment.

There is considerable fruitless discussion in the organizational literature of "goal-displacement," referring to what is perceived as a general tendency for organizations to turn away from their original goals. The problem with this kind of post hoc explanation is that, in many cases, the organizational analyst has all-too-naïvely accepted statements by officials as to what are organizational objectives. He has failed to recognize the fact that it is only after changes have taken place in the system that officials recognize these modifications and attempt to rationalize their behavior by making statements about changed organizational goals (Katz & Kahn, 1966).

A goal model of organizational evaluation also neglects the powerful influences of environmental factors. Negative environmental influences may make organizational goal-achievement extremely difficult, even though the organization is performing optimally. On the other hand, very positive environmental influences may assure significant goal-achievement in an organization which, on many criteria, would be considered to be performing quite poorly (Etzioni & Lehman, 1967).

Another problem with the goal model is the failure to recognize the existence of multiple goals. Acknowledging the difficulty in treating an organization as if it had a single goal or task, Rice (1963) cited the teaching hospital, prison and mental health service as particular examples of institutions which carry out many tasks simultaneously. Multiple goals are not necessarily compatible and involve competition for scarce resources by those subparts of the organization which are committed more to one goal than to others. For example, the mental hospital admits patients, provides therapy and custodial care for patients, attempts to place patients in the community, provides employment for mental health workers, looks after its employees, conducts research, keeps records and accounts and, if it has educational programs, provides professional training for nurses and residents. Usually, there is no settled priority of goals for such an organization. One of the goals becomes primary in the goal hierarchy at a given time, according to the balance of forces then operating. Failure to recognize the fact that such an organization has multiple goals and has to perform many tasks simultaneously may confound the assessment of organizational effectiveness. An evaluator is likely to encounter this pitfall by depending too much upon organizational spokemen's definitions of a single primary mission or task and because, as we noted above, particular goals are not recognized or even denied by organizational members.

What are the alternatives to the goal model of organizational achievement? One option is what we have been calling an "open system model." Rather than starting with the goal itself, this approach begins with an attempt to model the organization as a complex social unit which is capable of achieving goals or producing outputs. This model analyzes the relationships which must exist for the organization to operate at various levels of effectiveness and seeks to understand how the balance of relationships among the various component parts determine the outcomes of the total organizational system.

Etzioni & Lehman (1967) consider the "system-model" as clarifying a basic confusion that is difficult for the researcher to see or explain from a "goal-model" point of view. Applying a goal model, one is led to predict an increase in organizational effectiveness as more and more resources are committed to the goals of the organization. Mental health program analysis which is guided by a system model recognizes that an organization must allocate resources to activities other than those directly involved in goal-achievement and that there is a possibility of overallocation of resources to goal activities with the resulting effect of undermining activities necessary to maintain and integrate a complex organization which exists in an uncontrolled environment. Etzioni (1960) argues that organizational effectiveness must be considered in terms of an optimum distribution: "What counts is a balanced distribution of resources among the various organizational needs, not maximal satisfaction of one activity [p. 262]."

The goal model is simpler and less demanding of an evaluator than a system model, since the latter requires that an analyst, in addition to determining what goals an organization is pursuing, also acquire considerable information about the operating characteristics of the particular organization under study. Etzioni & Lehman (1967) describe the analyst's task as that of specifying what is a highly effective allocation of the organization's resources. Recognizing that the acquisition of information necessary to determine what is an optimum balance is likely to be quite demanding, they argue that "the efforts in obtaining the added indicators required for a *system-model* are not wasted, since the information collected in the process of developing a system model index will be of much value for the study of most organizational problems [Etzioni & Lehman, 1967, p. 8]."

Since goals are also an important part of a system model of organizational change, it becomes necessary to specify a general framework for goal-analysis consistent with the distinctive perspectives of such a system model. Four operationally different aspects of organizations are applicable to goal analysis in complex mental hospitals including: (1) environmental demands, (2) internalized personal goals, (3) perceptions of common organizational objectives and (4) allocated internal resources.

Environmental Demands

Social scientists have often noted that an organization's operational environment affects its goals, internal structure and processes. For example, Homans (1950) uses the concept of the "external system" to emphasize the shaping of the organization by its goals and environment. Thompson & McEwan (1958) stress the necessarily continuing interaction between an organization and its environment, resulting in a degree of environmental control over the organization. The products of the organization's activities or outputs must be acceptable and useful to some part of the organizational environment in order for the organization to have continued support from that part of the environment. Although goals grow out of an interaction between the organization and its environment, Thompson and McEwan point out that the organization is not necessarily without initiative in this process: "The differences between effective and ineffective organizations may well lie in the initiative exercised by those in the organization who are responsible for goal setting [p. 29]." Dill (1958) focuses on the relation of the environment to the organization by characterizing the input of information from the environment to which the organization might respond as the "task environment." He stresses the importance of differentiating between the environmental "demands" presented to a member of an organization and that person's recognition or interpretation of the stimuli. There is no necessary one-to-one relationship between environmental informational inputs and the cognitive formulations of goals developed by those role-incumbents in the organization who are exposed to such informational input from external sources.

In dealing with their external environments, organizations become differentiated into subsystems, each of which has as its major function the task of dealing with particular conditions in the environment (Rice, 1963; Lawrence & Lorsch, 1967). This results from the fact that each organizational unit has a capacity to deal with only a part of the total environment. The differential impact of environmental inputs provides different components of an organization with distinctive task demands as a result of the specific nature of environmental contacts, but as these inputs become internalized, they also affect the internal structure of the organization.

Lawrence & Lorsch (1967) have placed special emphasis on the states of differentiation and integration existing in an organizational system as these relate to particular economic and technical characteristics of the organization's environment. Limitations in the "span of surveillance" of any single group of managers cause organizations to divide into segments and units, each dealing with particular aspects of the internal environment. By unit differentiation, Lawrence and Lorsch mean "differences in goal orientation and in the formality of structure [1967, p. 10]." The concept of organizational differentiation is not new. However, earlier organizational theorists didn't recognize the systemic nature of organizations and failed to see that division of labor had consequences beyond the simple fact of segmentation; members of departments develop different attitudes and behavior patterns.

Internalized Personal Goals

Katz (1964), in reviewing the motivational basis of organizational behavior, concluded that the internalization of organizational objectives as part of an individual's own personal goals is generally confined to the upper ranks of managerial or executive personnel. He noted, however, that the internalization of total-system goals is found in voluntary organizations among personnel at lower levels of the organizational hierarchy as well. Two levels of organizational goals may be internalized by an individual. One type has to do with the objectives of the total system, a type often defined as the leadership's common goals. Another type of organizational goal which may be internalized by an individual consists of the goals and values of his personal subsystem, since they are more easily identified with than the overall objectives of the total system, particularly in a large multilevel organization where individuals at lower echelon levels may be removed from interaction with organizational leaders.

Goals are shared by group members, and the groups to which an individual feels commitment provide values against which he evaluates his own position and decisions. Merton (1957) has defined the "reference groups" to which an individual compares himself or to which he looks for normative standards as including both the groups of which the individual is a member as well as groups to which he does not belong but to which he orients himself in shaping personal behavior and evaluations. Focusing on the workers in a particular organization, two broad reference groups can be identified: (1) the work group and other subgroups within the focal organization, and (2) groups external to the organization. An individual's commitment to the internal and external groups may vary in degree and fluctuate over periods of time so that a reference group's power may vacillate accordingly.

Individual organization members tend to identify with organizational goals to the extent that they feel loyalty and commitment to internal work groups, and as these goals relate to those of powerful external reference groups such as professional societies. Professional workers in bureaucratic organizations have been extensively studied to test the hypothesis that such workers, identifying with multiple reference groups, are confronted with conflicting role-definitions and work-behaviors. A number of studies have found that professionals tend to develop either a "local" or "cosmopolitan" orientation. Those adopting the local pattern tend to be oriented to the internal work organization and give major consideration to its goals and expectations; those adopting a cosmopolitan orientation tend to give primary attention to the expectations and goals of external groups such as professional societies (Goldberg et al., 1965).

Perceptions of Common Organizational Objectives

Organizational goals can be defined as not only the commitments of individuals to the values of particular organizationally relevant groups, but also as the perception of the goals of executives who have major responsibilities to control and influence total organizational activities. Staff members may not always personally adhere to management's goals, but in a bureaucratic organization with a well-defined authority-system staff recognize that they are constrained by executive goals. Thus, it is important to not only consider the personal goals of staff but also to consider their perception of the goals of organizational leaders. An individual's perception of organizational goals may also be viewed as representing his view of the direction in which he thinks management would like the organization to go.

Allocated Internal Resources

When sociologists talk about organizational goals, they usually are referring to situations which do not yet exist but which are intended to be accomplished in the future by organizational activities. Following this model, one is put in the position of anthropomorphizing organizations if they indeed are to have intentions, or we must refer to the intentions of individuals which are somehow aggregated and identified as organizational goals.

Another approach to goal-definition involves an examination of the "primary task," which Rice (1963) has defined as the task that an institution was created to perform. Elaborating Trist Bamforth's (1951) concept of an enterprise as a "sociotechnical system," Rice emphasized the importance of examining the organization's commitment of both psychosocial and technical resources for the production of specific outputs in defining the primary task. As mentioned earlier, Rice, Trist and their associates at the Tavistock Institute of Human Relations over the years have continued to develop the model of a sociotechnical system which assumes that: (1) organizations are defined by their primary tasks; (2) organizations are open systems; and (3) organizations encounter boundary conditions which rapidly change the characteristics of the organization. This model incorporates the psychosocial aspects of goal-definition as well as the concept of allocating human and technological organizational resources for the production of specified outputs.

Integration and Coordination of the Internal System

We have previously noted the movement in open systems toward differentiated and elaborated subsystems. However, a system as a whole exists only to the extent that its parts continue to relate interdependently. Uncontrolled subsystem differentiation leads ultimately to divisiveness and a collapse of the whole. Integrative processes resulting in internal relations of cooperation among organizational subsystems, therefore, are a necessary aspect of systems-maintenance. This does not suggest that organizations have to be conflict-free for conflict and change are vital in a growing and adaptive system. It does emphasize, however, the need to insure the counteracting effects of integrating internal activities.

Early theorists, while not recognizing the open systems properties of organizations, did stress the need for organizational integration. Lawrence & Lorsch (1967) have observed that the early theorists tended to treat integration as a rational mechanical process which "would be taken care of simply by issuing orders through the management hierarchy, 'the chain of command [p. 12]." Later theorists focused on the resolution of differentiating conflict through the development of collaborative interpersonal relationships.

Rice (1963) and Haire (1959) have suggested that one of management's primary functions is the fostering of integration among organizational subsystems. As these subsystems respond differentially to environmental forces, management must provide integrative controls by bringing together representatives from competing organizational units, emphasizing their interdependence and personally making and implementing decisions clearly oriented to superordinate goals. We, thus, are suggesting that the integration of competing organizational units of departments depends upon management's ability to take an active role in determining overall policy. Without integrative activities leading to new states of dynamic, systemic equilibrium, there is a strong likelihood of organizational dissolution into unorganized components.

We must emphasize, however, that hierarchical relations are not the only formal channels of internal communication upon which an organizational system can build cooperative relations. While recognizing that those occupying roles high in the organizational hierarchy have particular leverage for the settlement of conflicts and can act as important symbols of systemic unity, Gross (1964) points out that modern organizations subdivide hierarchical authority and support the growth of a "multiple hierarchy" or "polyarchy." As a result, multiple authority channels cut across the multilevel organizational system. Informal communication channels, of course, are also a very important means of facilitating relationships that allow the efforts of individuals and organizational subsystems to be effectively coordinated.

The values and goals shared among organizational members, even when not overtly recognized, provide a binding force integrating organizational subparts. As we noted before, ideology, as a commonly adhered to system of ideas or beliefs, can serve as a rationale for the group's behavior and, thus, justify its position and policy. In organizations lacking clearly demonstrable and effective technology, commonly held beliefs about appropriate professional practice are particularly likely to play a significant role in molding systemic behavior.

ORGANIZATIONAL ADAPTATION AND THE ENVIRONMENT

If an organization is to exist as a distinct systemic entity, it must maintain discontinuity with its environment. This system "boundary" may be a territorial line. In a social system such as a human services organization, the boundary more importantly exists in "social space" as a discontinuity in patterns and clusterings of human activity. Thus, applying the term "system" to an organization implies interdependence in the sense that necessary input and output linkages are required in relation to other systems in the environment. However, "system" also implies independence in the sense that the organization acts to maintain the integrity of system elements through boundary control processes.

An organizational system may itself be viewed as playing a specialized role as a component or subsystem in a higher level suprasystem. The concept of environment and suprasystem should not be confused. The suprasystem of a focal system minus the system itself constitutes the immediate environment of the system. The entire environment of a system includes this immediate environment plus all the other suprasystems of which the focal system is a part, in addition to other systems at the same level with which it may or may not interact at any given time. In shifting focus from the level of the single organization to that of a complex network of organizations, there is strong appeal in speaking of a community suprasystem in which individual organizations constitute components or subsystems. From a general systems perspective, it is appropriate to apply the neutral terms of open systems theory and make cross-system-level generalizations, so long as it is recognized that the properties of a molar system may differ from those of a molecular system. However, as we attempt to talk about relationships among organizational systems, it is important that we note this latter qualification. As Gross (1966) has pointed out, larger and more differentiated interorganizational systems are likely to be marked by more complicated, divergent and conflicting roles and relationships than those found within a single organizational system.

As we noted before, a system at any level exists only to the extent that its parts or components are linked in a network of internal relations. Thus, as we begin to look at the relationships between a mental hospital and other community mental health resources, the "suprasystem hypothesis" must ultimately be tested empirically (Baker & O'Brien, 1971). The conceptualizing of a complex interorganizational system in which organizations exist as components or subsystems must be compared against the empirical evidence that such a macrosocial system does exist. Thus, the demonstration of component *interdependence* is a primary test of the empirical existence of a community suprasystem. Component interdependence is a measure of system cohesiveness, and may be defined as the extent to which a component depends upon other components as a source of inputs or decision premises, or as a receiver of a component's action. Although all organizational systems need not be assumed to be subsystems or components in some well-defined suprasystem, it is useful to conceptualize human service organizations such as mental hospitals as existing within a larger community suprasystem providing services responsive to the problems of people residing in a particular locality.

Change in Mental Health Organizational Systems

There are two major types of change in organizational systems—change in or among subsystems and change on the total system level. Total system change is usually examined in terms of change in output, whether this is deviation in values of a single output, or changes in the pattern or "mix" of outputs from the total organizational system. Subsystem change may or may not affect total system change as measured by deviations in output. For example, a mental hospital may undergo major changes at the level of roles or departments, but this may not be reflected in the output character of the total system.

Social systems can be examined and compared with regard to change from the perspectives of several different levels. For example, any particular organizational system can be evaluated in terms of its contributions to the superordinate systems of which it is a part. Clearly, the organization as a system must produce some important output for the suprasystem of which it is a part in order to receive, in turn, vital inputs. Thus, a mental hospital must produce outputs of a certain quality and quantity in order to continue receiving funds and legitimation from public sources. We have pointed out the relative advantages and disadvantages of considering an organizational system such as a mental hospital as part of a larger community mental health suprasystem. It also is important to remember that organizational systems vary markedly in their degree of interdependence, and that organizational interdependence is not necessarily symmetrical. However, whatever the nature of the interrelatedness between the organization and its environment, information about these relations provides a major means for assessing total system performance. Whether one looks at an organization as a relatively autonomous system or examines it from the perspective of the organization existing as a subsystem of a larger suprasystem, both approaches emphasize the importance of changes in the state of the organization vis-à-vis its environment.

It is not only the flow of outputs which portrays an organizational system's performance. All too frequently, the other major cyclic aspects of an open systems organization's functions are obscured. Input changes, or the resource-getting activities of an organization, as well as the resource-processing or throughput aspects of an organization, are equally important dimensions for assessing organizational performance. Yuchtman & Seashore (1967), opposing the usual overemphasis on evaluating change in organizational performance primarily on the basis of outputs, argue for a conception of organizational effectiveness based upon resource acquisition. Emphasizing the interdependence of the organization with its environment in terms of "transactions in which scarce and valued resources are exchanged under competitive conditions," Yuchtman & Seashore take the view that "the organization's success over a period of time in its competition for resources—i.e., its bargaining position in a given environment—is regarded as an expression of its overall effectiveness [1967, p. 891]." Clearly, then, change in an organizational system is multidimensional; the examination of change in any one part of the input-throughput-output cycle of organizational performance perforce involves an analysis of changes in other parts of these interrelated organizational activities.

Organizational change may be viewed as largely internally or externally induced. Reviews of the literature reveal no systematic empirical evidence on the relative influence of internal versus external factors in producing organizational change. In empirically examining specific organizational changes, it is important then to evaluate the relative influence of intrasystem and environmental antecedents of the change (Terreberry, 1968).

Another major dimension of organizational change is the degree to which it is passively adaptive or proadaptive. Organizational life consists of a series of necessary adaptations or adjustments within the system's operations so as to cope with internal and external demands. Since organizations are multilevel-multigoal systems, managerial subsystems are rarely in a position to have a full understanding of the total organizational situation. Nevertheless, organizations differ in the degree to which they have adequately developed specialized adaptive subsystems capable of assessing the internal and external environment and anticipating future organizational situations. Without such a specialized adaptive subsystem, the organization is constantly buffeted by unanticipated changes in the internal and external environment, with the result that the organization moves along erratically in one direction and then abruptly in another.

Organizations differ markedly in balancing their environmental relationships. Unlike business and industrial organizations, which function in a market situation where it is extremely important for survival to anticipate changes in consumer demand, human services organizations such as mental hospitals, until very recently, have tended to survive despite almost anything that they did. At times, the failures of the mental hospital and similar systems to meet demands of the larger society have been revealed through the efforts of energetic reformers in highly publicized exposes. However, it is only recently that mental hospitals, and other human services organizations, have become more directly accountable to citizens through the development of such mechanisms as citizen boards. Of course, mental hospitals had boards of trustees decades ago, but the trustee position often tended to develop into an honorific title rather than an active linkage role to the community. As strong constituencies, such as blacks and poor people, turn their attention to human service organizations, the mental hospital's survival will increasingly depend upon its ability to collect and evaluate information about its community's characteristics and needs. Much attention has been given in the hospital literature to the importance of internal communications, but communication is also very important as it provides channels for sensing external conditions and for impacting upon the community environment.

Burling and coworkers (1956) have noted, "Public relations are a two-way thing. The community presses in on a hospital in certain respects, and the hospital policies press back into the community to change its opinions and to create new ones." This give-and-take between an organization and its environment provides limits on the freedom of the hospital staff to act, and can either support or frustrate changing hospital goals. The attitudes and perceptions directed toward a mental hospital because of its past functioning continue unless they are actively changed by new organizational behavior-patterns. Unfortunately, however, certain new ways of functioning may be initially hindered and perhaps never allowed to develop because of the constraints imposed by longstanding community prejudices.

Despite the sanction given the mental hospital by outside systems such as state or federal government, the hospital may find its most difficult task to be that of legitimating a changed role in the community's human services system. Faced with the difficulty of relating to local health agencies at a time when they too are groping for new organizational missions, a changing mental hospital may find itself unduly confined by rational and coordinated planning models and thus decide to adopt a "go-it-alone" policy. That this development is already upon us can be seen in the growing number of neighborhood health centers, multiservice centers, etc., being created by different governmental branches to serve the same community without adequate attempts to coordinate their activities with each other or with already existing elements of the health and welfare network. For the community mental health program idea to work, more attention must be paid to breaking down through human linkages the barriers of inadequate communication and prejudice that block interorganizational cooperation. The hospital organizational system, both to anticipate changes in a community environment and to adapt its environment in light of internal changes in the organizational system, must develop adequate boundary-spanning roles. Thus, the examination of change in a developing mental hospital must focus on modifications in the internal system, shifts in the environment, and also transitions in the boundary-spanning structures and processes of the hospital.

SUMMARY

The functioning of mental health programs and related human services organizations can be best assessed

Table 4–1

Major Groups of Variables in Model of the Mental Hospital as an Open Organizational System

INPUT

- I. Patients
  - A. Demographic characteristics
  - B. Personal histories
- II. Staff and Students
  - A. Professionals, students and other personnel
    - 1. Professional skills, personality, attitudes, interests, goals, ideologies, habits, values, reference groups
- III. Legitimation
  - A. Political
  - B. Legal
  - C. Financial
- IV. Technology
- V. Material
  - A. Money
  - B. Supplies
  - C. Facilities

THROUGHPUT STRUCTURES

- I. Patient Care Subsystems
  - A. Patient admission
  - B. Therapy provision
    - 1. Verbal
    - 2. Somatic
    - 3. Activity
  - C. Custodial care provision
  - D. Community placement
- II. Training Subsystems
  - A. Education of professionals
    - 1. Residents
    - 2. Nurses
    - 3. Social workers
    - 4. Psychologists
  - B. Training of non-professionals
    - 1. Aides
    - 2. Other non-professional personnel
- III. Research Subsystems
- IV. Boundary-Spanning Subsystems
  - A. Aftercare
  - B. Primary prevention programs
  - C. Community relations
- V. Managerial & Administrative Subsystems
  - A. Receiving and processing information
  - B. Planning
  - C. Decision-making
  - D. Integrating
  - E. Controlling and directing
  - F. Personnel functions
  - G. Physical plant maintenance

OUTPUT

- I. Discharged Patients
- II. Trained or Educated Personnel
- III. Research
  - A. Information distributed
- IV. Change in Level of Health of the Population
- V. Patient Maintenance Programs
- VI. Community Education

FEEDBACK: Patients, other people, and information returned to the hospital from other systems in the environment.

through an open systems conceptual model. Within this framework, the mental hospital is considered as an open system composed of a set of human and material components grouped together into differentiated subsystems according to professional values and demands of the environment, and interacting with each other within a boundary which serves to separate the internal system from an external environment. As an open system, the mental hospital is defined by its inputs and outputs, i.e., its relationships with the environment.

The four interacting aspects of the mental hospital's organizational system which determine the state of the system at any given time are outlined in Table 4-1. These four basic dimensions are:

(1) Input—patients and staff and their demographic characteristics, personal histories, goals, ideologies, reference groups, abilities and habits, financial resources, legitimation, and technology.

(2) Throughput structures and processes— the internal operating and management subsystems of a hospital including departments, units and roles.

(3) Output— the numbers and types of patients who leave the hospital, the various trained students produced, research and other information distributed by the mental hospital organization.

(4) Feedback— the patients, other people and information which are shunted back to the hospital from other systems in the environment.

These four groups of variables are interdependent and must be considered collectively in evaluating the changing hospital organization.

The open systems model is concerned with establishing a working design of a social unit that is capable of achieving a variety of goals, such as patient care, research and training. Unlike the goal attainment model, the open systems assessment model seeks to determine the degree to which an organization realizes its goals under a given set of conditions. From this perspective, what counts is a balanced distribution of resources among all organizational objectives rather than the maximal attainment of a single goal. Thus, an organization cannot be considered as maximally effective if reorganization would improve a major subsystem without impairing other subsystems.

Change is evident in an organizational system when any aspect of the pattern for linking component parts undergoes major modification. When major internal structures, including informal structures and role patterns, undergo change, they are evaluated in this model as they affect the system's output mix. The organizational environments of mental hospitals, like other human services organization systems in this society, are increasingly turbulent. As a result, the hospital is increasingly less autonomous and organizational change increasingly tends to be externally induced. A hospital's success in obtaining needed supplies, providing services and surviving in a complicated environment depends upon its ability to develop internal subsystems which generate adaptive changes. Reactive internal changes to accommodate monetary environmental shifts are unlikely to be constructive in the long run and will result in the organization's disadvantage in meeting the demands of its input and output constituencies.

Employing an open systems model as a conceptual guide to organizational change is both complex and expensive. Obviously, the variety of interdependent variables which make up an organizational system is unusually diverse and even obscure. However, by considering the mental hospital and other human services organizations as a complex open people-belief-resource system, planners, administrators and researchers are better able to identify problems and formulate solutions.

Section II

Program Transition at the Mental Hospital

5. *Clinical and Administrative Organizational Patterns*

The initial section of this book has considered the historical and conceptual factors relevant during the past decade to mental health program development. Although the events of each passing year have continuously modified the relative impact of these factors, most mental health programs, and mental hospitals in particular, still function to a major extent within the previously described field of forces. We, therefore, will now examine the ways in which planning decisions, ideological commitments and conceptual orientations affect the mental hospital's efforts to join the mainstream of contemporary caregiving activities. Section II focuses upon the dynamic tensions associated with the struggle for organizational change by depicting the "state of a system" during an arbitrarily selected period of time. The intertwined dimensions of clinical practice and administrative structure in the changing mental hospital are considered in the following chapter, while the unique characteristics of these dimensions are analyzed in the subsequent chapters of Section II.

Earlier reviews of developing mental hospitals as systems, e.g., Perrow (1965) and Baker (1969), have drawn attention to the fact that complex organizations are the products of interaction between cultural and technological systems. Organizations are established on the basis of cultural values or ideological belief-systems which, within very broad limits, determine what their goals shall be. Techniques necessary to implement the goals are also supplied by the society, although a particular organization may develop new techniques or improve existing ones. Technology, in turn, influences structure, since a relevant organizational format is needed to accomplish given tasks. Only vague boundaries exist between the variables of goals, technology and structure because of their interdependency, and at any given point in time one variable may have the power to influence the others. Thus, the following description of a mental hospital as a system in flux is concerned with the institution's administrative patterns as a depiction of the management subsystems within which organizational tasks are performed, with its clinical services as a reflection of the conversion processes being utilized, and with the institution's community as an indication of the culture and values impacting upon hospital goals. The key role of the superintendent in the management subsystem, and his opportunities for guiding change, will be also considered.

STRAWS IN THE WIND

The period of the mid-1960s was marked by increasing national optimism about the mental hospital's viability. Many assumed that staff could move from a custodial to a treatment orientation, and that they could design treatment patterns adapted to the patient's rather than the institution's needs. By 1965, Boston State Hospital had already initiated organizational movement in keeping with these new directions, taking important strides toward a community mental health orientation even though it was still beset by a legacy of profoundly constraining problems (Schulberg & Baker, 1971). The hospital now operated a variety of intensive care subsystems designed to permit greater flexibility in meeting patients' needs. In addition to a reception service for acute inpatient care, the institution contained: a screening service which limited the residential stay for 20 percent of new admissions to less than three days; a series of day hospitals in different units of the acute and chronic services; and a specialized night hospital for longterm patients who had obtained community employment. Furthermore, a halfway house had been established on the edge of the hospital's grounds in the home formerly used by the superintendent, the foster family care program was growing, the home treatment service and the outpatient clinic continued to serve those who could be helped as outpatients, and a local child guidance clinic was developing closer ties to the hospital. The shift from a custodial to a therapeutic orientation could also be noted in the hospital's reduced inpatient census and the closing of several buildings which had been built early in the century. By late 1965, a census of the patients being treated by the hospital's many units revealed that 62 percent of the 3,045 individuals were inpatients while 38 percent were being treated in some form of outpatient care.

Improvement and growth do not occur, however, at a uniform rate in complex organizations with changing goals. Despite encouraging signs of movement, many formidable problems remained at Boston State Hospital. It was still faced with a tremendous backlog of chronic and geriatric cases. Of the hospital's 1,880 inpatients during October 1965, 54 percent had been institutionalized for more than five years and 46 percent were more than 60 years of age. In keeping with the public's negative image of mental hospitals, most of Boston State's 54 buildings had a drab, depressing, custodial aura which overwhelmed the serenity of the institution's 237-acre campuslike grounds. A company which considered producing a film about community psychiatry at Boston State Hospital decided to turn elsewhere since the poor image created by the physical facilities could overshadow programmatic accomplishments.

Staff perceptions of, and attitudes toward, organizational change are related to complex variables such as role and ideological commitment. Thus, it is no surprise that some key staff members were skeptical and even resistant to the notion of Boston State Hospital functioning in new ways. A family-oriented psychiatrist stated that even though the hospital's program in five years would have a community-based flavor with preventive services, in reality it still would be focusing primarily upon severely ill individuals. The new program directions also created a profound sense of uncertainty for several analytically oriented training psychiatrists, and they contended that change was occurring too rapidly. A social scientist on the scene contended, however, that the ripples of organizational change still were centered about the superintendent and that staff away from the vortex had been only dimly affected. Having assumed the superintendency in 1963, Dr. Greenblatt acknowledged in 1965 that his first two years had been spent "working from the outside in," but that now he was finally beginning "to get into the guts of the place . . . and would like to get deeper into the hearts of some staff people." He contended that almost all staff members could be induced to display initiative and creativity, and one technique for accomplishing this is to develop competitive situations. Thus, although the hospital's future character was still unclear, there could be little doubt that the superintendent was seeking to upset the organization's earlier equilibrium. If he was successful, new stability would have to be established since continuing tension among key personnel and the isolation of essential subsystems would adversely affect the hospital's ability to provide comprehensive services.

Administrative Patterns

Organizational theorists often assert that structure should follow function; i.e., administrative patterns should support programs and tasks rather than determining them. Although Dr. Greenblatt's conception of Boston State Hospital's mission differed from that of his predecessor and his initial actions had produced some loosening of the institution's organizational structure, the formal four-part divisional structure established in the 1950s still remained very much in evidence in 1965 (Table 5-1). The medical, professional services, nursing and administrative divisions had assumed new functions while continuing to perform old ones as well. Their formal interrelationships had adapted only minimally, however, to the superintendent's emphasis on revised organizational inputs and outputs.

Nevertheless, Belknap (1956) had noted in his classic study of Southern State Hospital's operational structure that the actual authority lines and functions of the system often depart widely from the formal table of organization, particularly when rapid program changes occur. A key task confronting the superintendent of an evolving mental hospital is that of designing a management subsystem which accommodates the needs of a burgeoning array of community-oriented services, those of existing profession-oriented divisions or those of both. The choice is affected by such factors as the priority to be assigned the new community services, and the potential for recruiting competent personnel in a highly competitive employment locale.

The superintendent of Boston State Hospital placed his initial priority upon recruiting and permitting creative staff members to enjoy maximum autonomy. As a result the home treatment service, the day hospital, the screening unit, the outpatient clinic, the aftercare program and the child guidance clinic performed deli-

TABLE 5–1
DIVISION STRUCTURE 1965

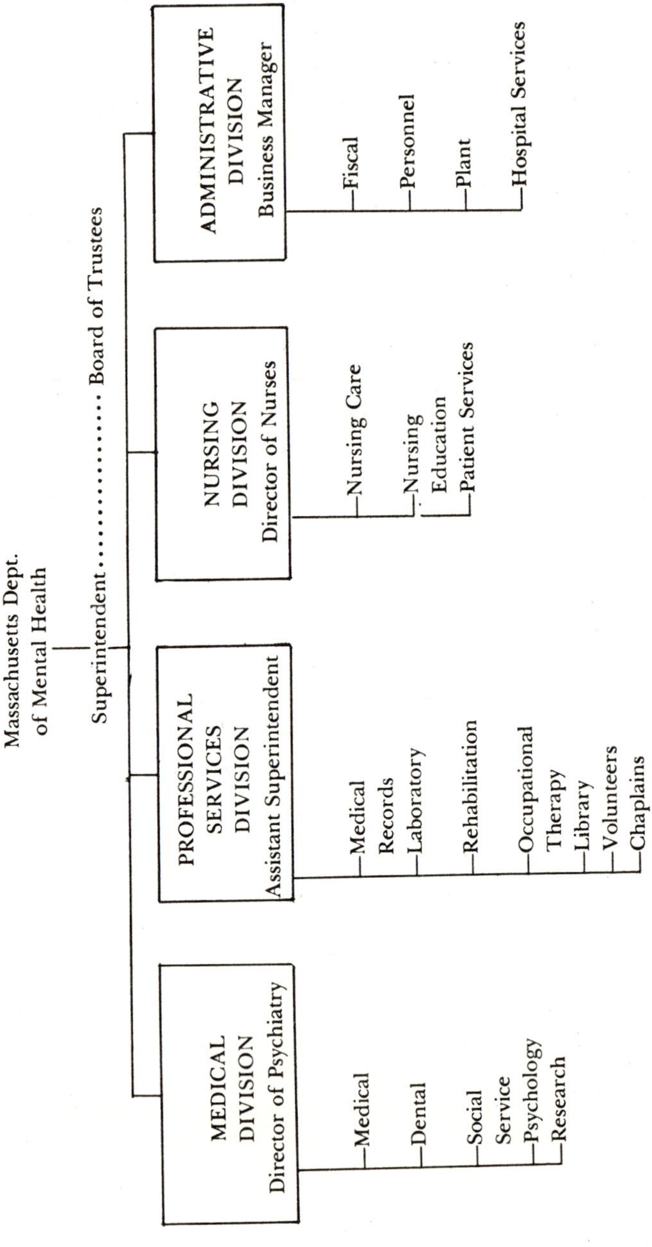

mited tasks, which by and large remained uncoordinated with either the hospital's inpatient subsystems or the community's larger caregiving network.

The mental hospital's growing community-oriented services generate highly visible dilemmas of integration, but their development provokes even broader systemic concerns. Changes are required in the institutions's entire administrative structure if it is to provide contemporary programs which are comprehensive and facilitate continuity of patient care. Thus, the superintendent of Boston State Hospital was confronted with the additional problems of how to realign long-standing relationships between the existing professional subsystems, and how to modify relationships within specific professional subsystems as program growth occurred. For example, conflicts between the medical and rehabilitation departments had been sparked by the efforts of the latter, supported by a 1964 NIMH Hospital Improvement Grant, to inject a work therapy orientation into the chronic wards. The psychiatrist directing one such unit commented derisively that "there are too many consultants around the Hospital and not enough staff to carry out the actual daily clinical work with patients." Treatment programs focused upon new approaches to patient care rather than professional prerogatives, provoked similar conflicts between rehabilitation counselors and occupational therapists, nurses and social workers, etc. Traditional domains were being trespassed, and agreement was needed on new administrative principles to guide interprofessional relations.

As programs change, working relations within the professional divisions similarly need reappraisal. New services for Boston State Hospital's chronic patients had produced many discharges and a lowered census on continued treatment units. The psychiatrists directing these units sought to expand their activities by accepting *selec-*

ted acute patients. The director of the reception service, while pleased to reduce his admissions load, strongly objected to the veto power which his colleagues sought to exercise. Interaction between these components of the medical division became increasingly tense, and new administrative guidelines were needed here as well.

The matter of where and how problems are to be resolved generates considerable concern, even controversy, within an organization when the decisionmaking processes are unclear or ineffectual. Such formal forums as the weekly psychiatric executive committee meeting, the weekly senior medical staff meeting and the monthly administrative staff meeting existed at Boston State Hospital, but there was considerable ambiguity as to the functions and powers of each of these groups. The senior medical staff viewed itself as impotent to affect basic policy changes since it perceived the administration as reserving for itself the prerogative of actual decisions. Conversely, the administration expressed impatience with the senior medical staff because of its alleged inclination towards talk rather than action.

It was within this setting of organizational anachronisms, changing professional roles and ambiguous working relationships that the unit system (Schulberg & Baker, 1969) received increasing attention as an administrative mechanism whereby the hospital could better assume its new mission of providing comprehensive, community-oriented services. The idea of decentralizing clinical services into administratively semiautonomous units was not a new one; it had been considered at various times during the previous decade. In the spring of 1965, three of the hospital's senior psychiatrists visited a number of unitized midwestern mental hospitals, and they returned as enthusiastic spokesmen for this approach. The administration decided that the staff's earlier objections to a unitized structure no longer existed, but the mechanical problems associated with implementing such a system were such that it would be more prudent to proceed with unitization in a stepwise rather than total fashion in order to rally maximum staff support. Regardless of the pace at which this change is undertaken, it nevertheless is clear that profound modifications result. Not only is the hospital's table of organization altered, but the structure of clinical subsystems and the role of professional departments are similarly affected.

Clinical Services

The establishment of a unit system requires a series of far-reaching administrative decisions about the programs and personnel to be affected by the reorganization. Mental hospitals with a complex array of clinical services, training activities and research programs are more difficult to unitize because of the disruptions to be imposed upon a myriad of well-established interaction patterns. Rather than leading to beneficial changes, the overwhelming anxiety unleashed by the staff's quest for new working relationships can possibly adversely affect patient care. The administrator must, therefore, be keenly sensitive to the subtle as well as overt forces at play within his organization as he designs and implements a unit plan. The nature of these complex patterns and their implications for a modified administrative structure will now be considered by analyzing Boston State Hospital's clinical, training and research subsystems as the relevance of unitization to contemporary goals is pondered.

Even though Boston State Hospital's 1965 administrative structure had remained largely unaltered since the mid-1950s, a variety of new clinical services had been added to the institution's therapeutic armamentarium during this decade. More patients could now be provided with continuity of care from preadmission to post-discharge, and the orientation in many wards had changed from custodialism to rehabilitation. Developments of this magnitude stem from many changes, including the institution's altered ideological climate and technological modifications.

The differences between a psychoanalytic and social-psychiatric approach to patient care have been outlined by Kotin & Sharaf (1967a), and these issues were brought into sharp relief by the superintendent's emphasis on reducing Boston State Hospital's census through whatever techniques possible. Ideological and therapeutic controversy, therefore, charged the scene. Analytically oriented staff members questioned the justification for assigning a very high priority to community placements for chronic patients since it was unclear that patients then adjusted better and/or were happier for it. The analysts emphasized that if you help patients look deeply into problems, environmental factors don't matter as much. On the other hand, staff with a social-psychiatric orientation considered psychoanalytic concepts appropriate for learning about schizophrenia but irrelevant to its treatment. They were irritated by the "bed rock analytic devotion to one-to-one relationships," and minimized the allegation that inpatients had been discharged prematurely or summarily. They contended that, on the contrary, inpatients were being taken advantage of for training purposes and being kept in individual therapy for prolonged periods of time; whatever spontaneous recuperative forces patients possessed were dissipated by the time they were transferred to a chronic service. In keeping with their emphasis upon returning the patient to the community as soon as possible, social psychiatrists utilized a variety of treatment modalities which inevitably clashed with those of psychotherapists.

An institution's effectiveness in providing individualized treatment and continuity of care, a key principle in community mental health programs, can be judged from the manner in which it organizes its inpatient services. Boston State Hospital's lingering adherence to less-than-optimal clinical practices, despite many advances, was seen in the fact that its inpatient services in 1965 still were operated as they had been for the previous two decades. All new patients were admitted to a central reception building to which a significantly large share of personnel were assigned since the aim was that of rapid patient discharge. Ratios of one nurse for every two patients and one psychiatrist for every 10 patients on the reception services contrasted sharply with ratios of only one nurse for every 10 patients and one psychiatrist for every 80–100 patients on chronic treatment units.

Despite this favored staffing pattern, the reception service's functioning remained less than optimal. The hospital admitted 2,000 patients per year, and this necessitated overly rapid turnover and insufficient attention to individual patient needs. The screening unit successfully diverted some admissions from the reception service but, like most mental hospitals, Boston State Hospital had developed few alternatives to inpatient care and admitted 90 percent of those appearing at its doors. As a result, the reception service's staff was worn down by the incessant pressure of quickly discharging or transferring recent admissions and often could not provide a high level of care. The "revolving door" thus became a major impetus to decentralize the hospital into semiautonomous units, each of which would treat acute as well as chronic patients.

We have noted earlier that the mental hospital's potential to function as an effective caregiving facility is dependent upon its ability not only to develop individualized treatment services for new patients, but also upon its success in generating alternative resources for the overwhelming number of chronic residents which it has accumulated over the years. Despite the minimal resources devoted to the care of these patients, assigned staff and funds still represent a significant drain upon the hospital's limited assets. In contrast to the unchanged, problematic nature of the reception service, major modifications had occurred within Boston State Hospital's continued treatment service. Housed in a series of older structures, the service over the years had developed a reputation as a "hot bed of custodialism and one of the original snake pits." By September 1965, however, the service's peak census of 1,000 had been reduced to 400; some of the early twentieth-century buildings had been closed, and an air of optimism and excitement marked the activities of many new staff members.

The discharge of as many chronic patients as possible to a variety of community settings had become the staff's major goal, and they concentrated on developing alternative resources to hospitalization. A family-care program was initiated and after a period of difficult recruitment problems, enough local families were located to care for almost 100 patients. Another major strategy for reducing the service's census was to transfer chronic and aged patients to nursing homes. Stotsky (1966) reported that 141 such patients were transferred during the period of July 1963–June 1964; and only 20 returned to the hospital within six months of placement. However, this tactic generated considerable opposition, and staff questioned whether it was appropriate to transfer chronic patients who had become well adjusted to the hospital's custodial environment to a setting providing even less psychiatric care. Despite the skepticism of local professionals, the service's success in rehabilitating many supposedly unmovable chronic patients ultimately gained national recognition in a *Saturday Evening Post* article about mental hospitals (Martin, 1968).

In addition to the several inpatient units which the mental hospital operates for its acute and chronic patients, subsystems of varied elaboration have emerged over the years to meet the needs of special groups like adolescents, the aged, the physically ill, alcoholics, etc. The linkages between these special subsystems and the other inpatient units may range from the highly structured to the purely informal, and represent a further factor to be dealt with in reorganizing the hospital's clinical services into a comprehensive program. Some institutions prefer to maintain specialized patient-care subsystems, since their clinical activities are deemed to be unique. Other mental hospitals are primarily concerned with integrating care for all residents of given geographic areas within a single unit and discourage specialized subsystems. These differing approaches affect the mental hospital's ability to achieve an integrated approach to comprehensive services, as can be seen in the diverse strategies guiding Boston State Hospital's evolving geriatric and adolescent services.

Approximately 25 percent of Boston State Hospital's admissions were over age 60, and since the early 1950s they had been treated on the geriatric pavilion or on the medical-surgical service. From 40 to 50 percent of these individuals subsequently were released to the community, but despite efforts to provide necessary medical and psychiatric attention, almost one third of the admissions died within 12 months of hospitalization (Stratton & Barton, 1964). The director of the geriatric service concentrated on consolidating the program components into a single building, and he concluded in his 1964 annual report that the major emphasis must be directed toward lowering the service's census by improving its release rate. The priority, therefore, was to be upon the treatment of acute geriatric patients by developing specialized services within the hospital and in the community since it was felt that the aged received insufficient attention within general caregiving resources. A separate day care program and geriatric aftercare service were organized, and it was hoped that improved continuity of care would minimize hospitalization. Help was also expected from the recently passed Medicare legislation which could provide up to $1.5 million in federal funds for the hospital's 700 patients over age 65. Thus, the director of geriatric services was optimistic that his program would improve with the centralization of a comprehensive hospital treatment subsystem for the aged.

That the changing mental hospital can also take a decentralized approach to meeting the unique clinical needs of certain populations is evident in program strategies for emotionally disturbed adolescents. Their treatment has long been problematic because of the troublesome management issues associated with their care. Previous organizational solutions have included the admission and treatment of only special cases, and/or the development of a special adolescent unit with unusually high staff-patient ratios. The former approach is contrary to the spirit of a comprehensive mental health program, while the latter is extremely difficult to achieve in institutions which have many clinical services competing for limited resources. The rapid growth in Boston State Hospital's adolescent admission rate forced it to seek other alternatives. A small Adolescent Service was organized early in 1965 to provide consultation and special services for these patients, who continued to reside on wards scattered throughout the institution where their physicians retained primary responsibility for their care. Initial success with this consultation model led the service to expand its efforts and by late 1965, it sought to include every hospitalized adolescent within its program. The service's staff contended that it could combine special educational and recreational facilities for adolescents with routinely available ward resources so that mental hospitals economically could meet this group's unique inpatient needs (Kris & Schiff, 1969). If this was to be a successful treatment model, a new amalgam of hospital subsystems would have to be forged by combining centralized and decentralized resources.

This overview of the varying rates at which program development occurs at an evolving mental hospital, and the administrative complexities associated with this progress, makes it clear that significant changes in the intake policy and treatment activities of any single subsystem also affect the clinical services and administrative structure of other patient-care subsystems. Thus, regardless of which organizational strategy is adopted for integrating patient-care activities, the solution will affect the plans and aspirations of all hospital divisions and programs. They, in turn, must devise new modi operandi for retaining internal cohesiveness and effective linkages to the institution's other subsystems.

TRAINING AND RESEARCH PROGRAMS

A complex organization is committed to the fulfillment of many goals beyond its most obvious ones so that intricate balances must be established among program priorities and in resource-allocations. Etzioni (1960) has noted that excessive organizational success in achieving some goals may paradoxically produce failure in achieving others. In the mental health field, psychiatric institutions perform many functions in addition to patient care.

Training and research programs often complement the institution's clinical purposes, but in some instances are competitive with and overshadow patient activities. Staff conflict may then ensue unless administrators explicate organizational priorities and justify resource deployment. The evolving mental hospital often pursues its new goals through multiple program modalities, with the rationale that expanded training and research activities support high-level clinical services. The powerful influences exerted upon organizational development by the structure and philosophy of the training and research subsystems can be seen in a review of their salient characteristics at Boston State Hospital.

Training Programs

Opportunities for the basic training of several mental health disciplines had existed for many years at Boston State Hospital, and during the 1960s the institution had expanded into such diverse areas as advanced residency training in community psychiatry and "careers in mental health" for high school students. The superintendent asserted that, in point of fact, the hospital actually was a training center serving broader educational functions than many of the prestigious local academic centers. Nevertheless, it was also clear that the training program for psychiatric residents had the highest priority and was of greatest concern to the administration and senior staff. The superintendent stated in a 1965 interview, "This is a medical organization and from the training of psychiatric residents, the whole thing takes its tone. We could be successful in every other area, but if we were unsuccessful in that it would leave a tremendous gaping hole."

Within a small and selective training institution, there is little doubt that the resident's educational needs have the highest organizational priority and, therefore, determine related policy. Within the large mental hospital, however, this high level of priority is more difficult to agree upon and implement, and friction ensues between clinically and educationally oriented personnel. The steps taken by Boston State Hospital to insure the success of residency training efforts cogently indicate the dilemmas facing the mental hospital as it strives to balance the competing or complementary needs of training and service, as well as to affect the transition from a narrow psychoanalytic orientation to a broader community mental health perspective.

As Boston State Hospital's focus in 1965 increasingly centered upon rapid patient discharge and reduction of the census, the clinical demands upon staff grew and the psychiatric residents were forced to become more actively responsible for service needs. Complaints were expressed that the training of residents was being overlooked in the face of clinical pressures and that supervisory arrangements were inadequate. Some senior psychiatrists maintained that earlier Boston State Hospital residents knew that the staff's major allegiance was to their training, and that recruitment problems would arise in the future if residents felt they were being submerged in the hospital's turbulent efforts to redirect treatment programs. Administration attempts to meet resident dissatisfaction ranged from immediate steps to insert greater structure into the existing training to a reemphasis on the resident's primary role as student rather than service-provider.

Nevertheless, not only did the structure of the residency training program and its organizational priority remain at question, but the program's very purpose also became a source of controversy. In the past, there had been agreement that residency training should emphasize a psychoanalytic orientation and prepare the residents to practice individual and group psychotherapy.

The new superintendent, however, placed greater weight upon eclectic concepts and favored community-oriented social-psychiatric treatment measures.

The possibility of the hospital adopting the unit plan brought these differing emphases into sharper focus. If the hospital was decentralized, residents would spend greater lengths of time on a given service and their exposure to varied orientations would be limited even further. A clinical director contended that the training received under the unit system would be excellent for those psychiatrists seeking careers in mental hospitals but not for the vast majority whose ultimate aim was private practice. Since many other local training centers would continue, as before, to prepare their residents for private practice, a change in Boston State Hospital's organizational structure and conceptual emphasis would place the institution at a disadvantage in recruiting top-level residents.

The superintendent and others heatedly disputed the contention that residents should be trained to offer two kinds of treatment, the first for hospital patients and the second for private ones; psychiatrists should be able to function in all settings. Again, however, the dispute about residency training was reflecting basic staff differences as to the hospital's overall purposes and the procedures for achieving them. It was also clear that the institution's training and clinical subsystems were closely interwoven and that the unique needs of each subsystem would both abet as well as constrain efforts to produce organizational change.

Research Activities

In addition to clinical services and training programs, research activities are another significant function vying for organizational priority and a share of the mental hospital's limited resources. Although the magnitude of research endeavors varies considerably among institutions, there is a generally shared feeling among administrators of dynamic, progressive organizations that research contributes in a major way to maintaining a professionally stimulating and clinically rewarding environment. As mental hospitals have sought to gain a vibrant role in community mental health networks, they frequently have undertaken research and demonstration projects as vehicles for attracting competent staff, for raising staff morale and for standardizing erratic clinical practices. From the research director's vantage point, Rapaport (1968) has described a balanced mental hospital research program as including longterm investigations which contribute to the reservoir of fundamental knowledge as well as studies of daily crises and patient-management problems of immediate concern to clinicians and administrators.

Research studies had been conducted at Boston State Hospital for several decades, but they assumed a new importance and centrality when Dr. Greenblatt, himself an experienced researcher, assumed the hospital's superintendency. He considered a major research program to be an excellent means for strengthening institutional pride and raising additional funds, and senior clinicians and department heads were prodded to develop projects which could attract federal and foundation support.

In the fall of 1965, the hospital published a directory of research activities which included descriptions of 19 projects of varying scope and complexity. The hospital's research program included projects of both shortterm as well as longterm significance, and generally reflected eclectic, social-psychiatric interests rather than the psychodynamic concerns of analytically oriented clinicians. Research reports were becoming accepted as a legitimate organizational output along with discharged patients and trained personnel. Some staff members even felt that higher status could be obtained within the hospital's hierarchy if one's salary was supported by special research funds rather than the hospital's regular budget.

Along with these developments, however, concern was also being expressed by key staff about an excessive emphasis upon research. They contended that research was disrupting existing working patterns and diverting limited resources from clinical functions, conflicts that Almond & Kupfer (1969) and Jacobs & Kotin (1972) have found to be typical within complex psychiatric institutions with a strong research orientation. A widely shared skepticism also existed about the utility of research findings. For example, Grinspoon, Ewalt, & Shader's (1968) study demonstrating the relative inefficacy of psychotherapy with chronic schizophrenics was discussed by the senior staff, and they doubted whether controlled research really could investigate the salient processes and outcomes of this therapeutic modality. The staff concluded that although individual psychotherapy might well be ineffective with chronic schizophrenics, nevertheless it should be continued since the experience was helpful in teaching residents the nature of schizophrenia. Thus, research studies were an expanding hospital function with increasing prestige, but they also were creating tension among staff whose previous work patterns and organizational relationships were being upset.

The Hospital's Environment

It is clear that no caregiving organization can remain viable and relevant if it functions as a closed, self-contained system. The organization must interact with its environment in multiple ways at a variety of systems levels if it is to maintain necessary sanctions for programs, inputs for activities and a market for products. However, interaction and relations with the environment are affected by numerous factors over which the organization exerts only varying degrees of control. For example, the mental hospital can manifest considerable influence over its staff's interaction patterns with local agencies so that it may deliberately determine relationships with the community's caregiving network. On the other hand, the institution has relatively little control over the profound fiscal decisions reached at the more distant level of state and federal systems which affect its funding and budget. The factors affecting a community-oriented mental hospital's efforts to expand environmental linkages and to relate to appropriate citizen and caregiving systems will now be considered.

The Catchment Area

The delineation of appropriate geographic entities to be served by urban mental health programs has been fraught with difficulties. In many parts of the country relevant sociopolitical criteria often cannot be accommodated within the federal guidelines which impose population limits of approximately 75,000 to 200,000 people upon the catchment area. Nevertheless, regardless of how artificial or meaningful the resulting boundary lines, mental hospitals must be knowledgeable about the unique characteristics of the catchment areas assigned to them if they are to assume expanded, community-oriented roles. The catchment area's historical roots, ethnic composition, socioeconomic makeup, political structure, etc., are among the forces affecting the caregiving network in general, and the psychiatric institution in particular, as they seek to fulfill critical functions.

For many years Boston State Hospital had been legislatively mandated to serve the entire city of Boston. An analysis of the hospital's clientele in the fall of 1965 revealed that indeed inpatients originated from throughout the city, with a disproportionately high number from lower socioeconomic sections and an underrepresentation from the more affluent neighborhoods. In contrast, the hospital's outpatient programs primarily were serving residents of those geographic sections physically close to the institution.

The definition of the community to be served by Boston State Hospital was altered by the 1965 statewide plan for expanded community mental health programs (Massachusetts Mental Health Planning Project, 1965). The plan drastically reduced the hospital's longstanding, overburdening mission to serve all of Boston and assigned it a more limited catchment area (Figure 5–1). The change from providing comprehensive services for 650,000 people to only 230,000 clearly was one of the most helpful political decisions since the Commonwealth's early-1900s policy assigned the hospital responsibility for the entire city. The implications of this change confronted Boston State Hospital in late 1965. Above and beyond the new clinical programs which would be made possible by a reduced admissions load, the delimited catchment area also would make it possible for the hospital to become involved in its community's social problems if it believed that the causative factors of mental illness were related to environmental factors. Alternatively, it could continue viewing the individual patient as the focal unit for study and treatment, with his community of origin as a background of secondary significance.

Varying conceptions of a mental hospital's appropriate involvement with its community are of practical as well as theoretical importance, particularly when the catchment area is in the midst of turbulent change. Although

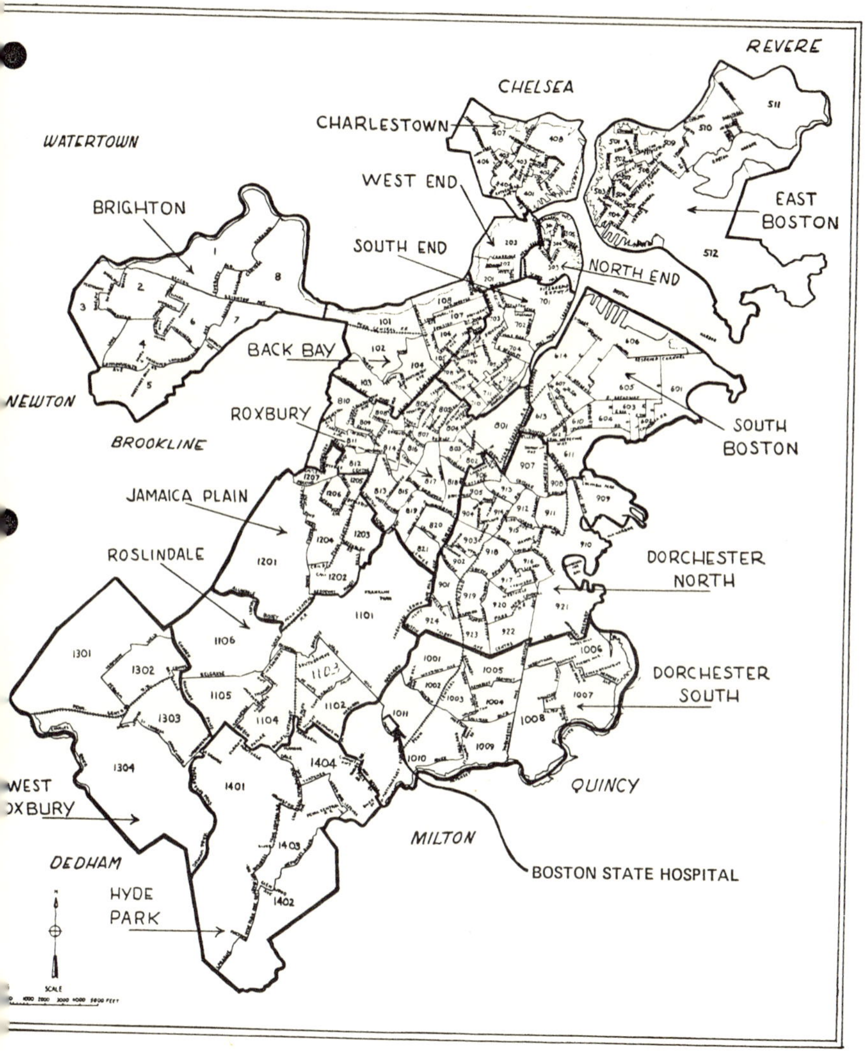

Fig. 5–1

City of Boston

the total population of the catchment area served by Boston State Hospital had increased by only 4% between 1960 and 1965, the ethnic and racial composition of its residents was changing markedly. The neighborhood where the hospital was physically located and in which it had previously developed the bulk of its community services had been predominantly Jewish but now was rapidly becoming black. The area's main thoroughfare was later described as a mixture of synagogues and soul shops, kosher butchers and realtors; fear of black teenage crime crippled the whites too old or too poor to move, and police protection occupied people's minds (*Time*, April 6, 1970). The public school system and other social resources were also affected by these population changes so that a variety of challenges faced the hospital's staff if it wished to immerse itself in the social crises of its immediate community.

Citizen Links

As the mental hospital seeks to expand its community-oriented services and to forge new linkages with the residents and caregivers of the area, it often finds that its efforts are constrained by the institution's public image and by previous relationships with local resources. Interviews with staff at local health and welfare agencies and with the editors of community newspapers frequently reveal that earlier negative stereotypes are still prevalent, particularly among those individuals having minimal contact with the institution. For example, when the director of a nearby alcoholism sanitarium described Boston State Hospital as doing "great work," he was referring to the carnivals and other social activities held to make patients' lives easier. Thus, people's perceptions of the mental hospital's caregiving role continued to be flavored by an awareness that custodial activities dominated programs and that admissions were often terminal in nature.

Despite widespread pessimism and misconceptions, various community-oriented activities can begin to alter the hospital's image. Public relations efforts by Boston State Hospital in the late 1950s had gained the local merchants' acceptance for an open-door policy, and the animosity of nearby residents had been reduced. A public relations expert had been hired with federal funds earlier in 1965 to upgrade the institution's public image. The tenor of newspaper publicity was shifting from the sensationalism of the past to constructive descriptions of the hospital's extensive efforts to produce change. In particular, the home treatment service's widespread involvement with general practitioners and visiting nurses had earned new respect for the hospital's ability to provide high-quality services.

The numerous volunteer groups regularly visiting the mental hospital constitute an additional community link. These citizen groups range from the representatives of churches and synagogues fulfilling a traditional charitable role to sophisticated individuals seeking the opportunity personally to provide chronic patients with a warm human relationship. A fall 1965 conference at Boston State Hospital on the volunteer's role (Ewalt, 1967) attracted more than 200 participants.

One of the oldest, and yet most quixotic, links between the mental hospital and its community is the citizen's role as advisor or trustee to the institution. Both parties recognize their need for and responsibility to each other, and yet the relationship often remains desultory and irrelevant. A board of trustees had been established by state statute in the early 1900s to oversee Boston State Hospital's patient-care activities. Over the years, however, this responsibility most often was expressed through concern for the plant's physical condition, whose improvement or deterioration could easily be assessed, rather than by involvement with the abstract details of program development. Although effective as a legislative lobbying group and genuinely determined to improve the physical and clinical conditions under which patients were treated, the board generally was unfamiliar with the emerging psychiatric ideology of the 1960s and continued to reflect through its deliberations a lingering concern with custodial activities. Furthermore, the Board's members consisted of individuals who had received longterm political appointments from the governor. The prevailing sentiment of the mid-1960s, however, favored "maximum feasible participation" by local residents on policymaking bodies. Thus, the board of trustees originally designed to insure the mental hospital with citizen input and involvement had become anachronistic in composition.

Movement into the era of community mental health has led to questioning not only the membership of hospital-community citizen bodies but their structure and functions as well. The Community Mental Health Acts passed by Massachusetts and other states in the mid-1960s sought to give newly established citizen boards wider authority for program analysis and budget review. The full extent of these responsibilities remained ambiguous, however, and the personnel to help fulfill them nil. Thus, Boston State Hospital was faced in 1966 with the prospect of having to relate to its traditional Board of Trustees, as well as to a newly mandated Area Board whose philosophy would be community-oriented but whose demands could be controversial.

In general, then, the hospital had become quite sophisticated in techniques for involving local citizens as volunteers providing a variety of crucial services. Citizens could successfully be induced to donate their personal labor, to supply the hospital with equipment unavailable through the state budget, and to provide chronic patients with invaluable warm human contacts. Less expertise and motivation were evident among hospital personnel, however, in devising methods for involving local citizens in policy and program decisions. The professionals recognized that citizens could make significant contributions toward upgrading clinical services, but wished to reserve for themselves the ultimate decisions about how, where and when this was to be done.

The Caregiving Network

The third environmental variable of significance to the community-oriented mental hospital is the caregiving network of which it is a component. The complexity of the network and the relationships of participating members vary over time in accordance with changing social policy, intake practices, fiscal needs, technological advances, personnel standards, etc. As comprehensive community mental health programs have evolved in recent years, their interorganizational structures resemble either the medical-organizational or human services networks, with psychiatric facilities assigned differing roles and responsibilities in each (Schulberg, 1969). In either of these networks, however, the mental hospital's ability to generate appropriate inputs and outputs is significantly enhanced or constrained by the interaction patterns which it establishes with other community resources participating in the care of the mentally ill. Thus, mental hospital personnel clearly recognize the need for improved linkages among themselves and local resources if their facility's inpatient census is to be reduced and the caregiving burden is to be equitably shared.

Procedures for achieving these goals are less obvious, however, and mental hospitals have experimented with various clinical and administrative alternatives. At Boston State Hospital, staff experiences with the community's resources had been limited to that of hospital boundary-spanning services like the foster family program and the home treatment service. By 1965 an increasing number of hospital psychiatrists began to recognize that sophisticated resources existed outside of their own institution. Despite this attitudinal shift, however, most hospital personnel still found it more practical and congenial to invite community caregivers into the hospital than to venture personally into the unfamiliar environs of their institution. Consequently, the staff continued to focus predominantly upon the dynamics and treatment of individual patients, perhaps through improved liaison with other agencies, and not upon the management of broader social problems affecting the mental health of local residents. The interaction pattern with other community resources thus was moving in the direction of an effective medical organizational network, within which the hospital could play a central role in coalescing community resources to care for the catchment area's acutely and chronically mentally ill. The idea of expanding into broader human services, relating to educational and recreational agencies, and focusing upon preventive activities in addition to clinical programs was alien to most of the hospital's staff.

THE SUPERINTENDENT'S QUEST FOR CHANGE

Any analysis of organizational change must consider the nature of the management subsystems guiding program development. The role of the chief executive is particularly crucial in this subsystem since he sets an ideological tone and operational pace central to the direction and speed of program change. The superintendent of the mental hospital exerts inordinate influence on the priorities and services of his institution since he statutorily is vested with the responsibility for all that transpires within his domain, a responsibility which often has produced conservative rather than daring administrative styles. Belknap (1956) described the newly appointed mental hospital superintendent as having been traditionally faced with the dilemma of whether to accept the institution's services and structure as he found them, and thus continue adequate but custodial services; or whether to abandon traditional routines, install modern psychiatric practices and thus create administrative turmoil. His choice of the former alternative was reinforced for many years by the ambiguity of societal concern for the mentally ill.

In recent years, however, it has become obvious that despite lingering ambivalences as to the goals, techniques and locations of mental health services, the superintendent of a mental hospital must stimulate the movement of his institution toward community mental health programs if it is to survive. Accepting this mandate, the superintendent must choose and implement a strategy for promoting maximal change and minimal confusion, an undertaking fraught with dilemmas at all points in the process. Hirschowitz (1971) has described the "promotion or commotion" pitfalls to be avoided by the leader of a community mental health program, and the need to utilize a variety of administrative, organizational, managerial, negotiating and political skills in pursuing program goals. The leader must be particularly adept at distinguishing between economic, political and social power-sources as new relationships are developed within his institution, and between his institution and its environment.

The complex interplay of management change strategies and the institutional forces striving for homeostasis can be seen in Dr. Greenblatt's efforts as superintendent to move Boston State Hospital toward community mental health organizational goals and activities. Perceiving the development of institutional pride and prestige to be the most pressing need, Dr. Greenblatt devoted his initial two years as administrator to establishing research and demonstration programs in the belief that such ventures were optimal vehicles for strengthening staff morale and self-respect. Utilizing his extensive familiarity with university research ventures, the superintendent attracted several prominent investigators and teachers so that an academic-like environment began to emerge on the hospital's campus.

From a systems perspective, however, the organization must concern itself with insuring an optimal distribution of limited funds and personnel among equally pressing needs in the areas of patient care, research and training. Since agreement on the optimal blend rarely is forthcoming among competing interests, particularly when ideological differences exist, a struggle may ensue between the administrator and key organizational participants (Kotin & Sharaf, 1967a). At Boston State Hospital, many individuals were distressed by what they perceived to be the superintendent's overemphasis on training and research to the detriment of patient care. A member of the hospital's board of trustees indicated that his group's key job was to make sure that patients received good care, that the buildings were in good condition, and that wards were kept clean. He feared that these vital functions had assumed a secondary importance in 1965 because of the superintendent's other interests. Dr. Greenblatt's repeated assertions that service was his highest priority, and that good training and research supported this end, failed to convince the disbelievers.

An administrator's success depends not only upon his proper juggling of program goals but also upon his managerial techniques for implementing them. In mental hospitals striving for new program directions, the superintendent must make the key decision about the rapidity with which change can occur (Greenblatt, Sharaf, & Stone, 1971). Dr. Greenblatt thought that he had to create a fast thrust if Boston State Hospital was successfully to compete for scarce resources, and he, therefore, utilized what Kotin and Sharaf (1967b) have described as a "loose administrative style." Deeming rigid hierarchical structures to be counterproductive in certain instances, the superintendent bypassed supervisory channels and frequently assigned to capable junior staff senior, perhaps even controversial, responsibilities.

The disruption of established bureaucratic routines inevitably produces dismay, even hostility, among affected personnel. Dr. Greenblatt was perceived by many of his staff as seeking change for the sake of change, as acting impulsively and even autocratically and failing to appreciate the hospital's needs as a total system. The superintendent, however, viewed his role as that of producing consensus for the maximum degree of disequilibrium tolerable to the institution as it undertook new program directions. Thus, by late 1965 the superintendent had conveyed his priority for a hospital ethos in which change is highly valued. In addition to furthering research and training activities, Dr. Greenblatt was ready to turn his attention to the reorganization of clinical services on the basis of the unit system. The impending changes were welcomed by those seeking the introduction of community-oriented programs and the modification of existing emphases on acute patient care. This new hospital culture was less acceptable, however, to those concerned with maintaining earlier professional standards, particularly in the area of training. Their discomfiture was intensified by the superintendent's unique administrative approach to problem-solving.

SUMMARY

Like most complex organizations which experience difficulty in simultaneously fulfilling a multitude of functions, the mental hospital in 1965 was beset by troublesome problems which had to be resolved if it was to function effectively as a community mental health center. The backlog of chronic patients had been reduced through intensive rehabilitation efforts and extended linkages to community resources, but the management of an overwhelming inpatient admissions load still required improvement. A variety of services had been developed to treat outpatients living in the community but these programs generally functioned in isolation from the hospital's major inpatient units. In institutions like Boston State Hospital, training and research increasingly competed with clinical services for prestige and scarce resources, and the feeling was growing that patient care was suffering as a result. It was also becoming apparent that some new state community mental health acts, through which the hospital would be assigned a much more delimited catchment area, could produce major changes in the hospital's basic character. A decision would have to be made whether to continue focusing primarily on clinical activities and individual patients, or whether also to become involved with the catchment area's social problems as they relate to mental illness.

6. *Unitizing the Mental Hospital*

In spite of widespread pessimism about the mental hospital's role in community mental health activities, fiscal and legislative developments in the 1960s led to consideration of the facility's potential contribution to comprehensive programs. If mental hospitals were to act upon this revitalized franchise, it was clear that they must modify their administrative and clinical structures to better fulfill contemporary, societally determined tasks. The overwhelming size of institutions, in terms of both their thousands of patients and staff as well as their vast physical plants, frequently had produced a stultifying organizational model in which centralized, hierarchical control was maintained over virtually all of the institution's internal and external activities. The model had reinforced the mental hospital's traditionally insular character, the deployment of resources in favor of the acutely ill to the detriment of chronic patients, and the thwarting of initiative and creativity among those so bold as to seek modifications in the institution's priorities and operating procedures. Thus, it was clear that for the mental hospital to assume contemporary functions, it must establish administrative structures which accommodate traditional intraorganizational priorities like acute inpatient care while simultaneously fulfilling societal demands for community-based services.

As organizations have grown in size and complexity, decentralization has been utilized as an administrative strategy for coping with emergent problems. In a pioneering effort back in 1920, General Motors was reorganized so that daily operating responsibilities were assigned to the divisional level, whereas longterm decisions and interdivision coordination were handled at headquarters. Pervading this design were the concepts of clear definition of authority and responsibility, and carefully developed systems of information flow to insure control and coordination.

Decentralization, as a strategy for coping with changing needs, has been thought to produce any, or all, of these benefits: giving autonomy to the work level at which organizational goals can best be operationalized; permitting problem-solving through prompter and more knowledgeable action; allowing greater organizational flexibility in transactions with the environment; requiring less complicated and precise systems of organizational coordination; and creating a more personal social climate for lower-level managers and workers because of the more meaningful roles assigned to them. Along with the benefits of decentralization, it also has been recognized that if a viable system is to be maintained, special effort is required to integrate the decentralized components. The organization as a whole can exist and be effective only to the extent that autonomous subsystems relate to each other, and a proliferation of uncontrolled subsystems will lead to divisiveness and ultimately organizational dissolution.

DECENTRALIZING THE MENTAL HOSPITAL

Belying the frequent contention that research has little impact on practice, it is clear that studies of the mental hospital as an organization or community (e.g. Belknap, 1959; Caudill, 1958; Stanton & Schwartz, 1954) were instrumental in highlighting the manner in which organizational characteristics affect treatment practices and patient care. These studies emphasized the need to modify such problematic practices as confused channels of authority and responsibility, opposing therapeutic orientations among different categories of personnel, sharply fixed roles in the status hierarchy and limited communications between patients and staff. Given the mental hospital's problem of managing large blocks of patients with small groups of supervisory personnel, the bureaucratic structure inevitably had led to alienation between patients and staff (Mirelowitz, 1972).

Along with the attention focused upon the authoritarian, dehumanizing practices evident in the large mental hospital, there also emerged proposals for democratic, therapeutically oriented programs (Jones, 1953) which would necessitate reorganization of the hospital into smaller, more manageable units. Although the motive of establishing a therapeutic community is not always behind the efforts to restructure a hospital, the issues raised by this clinical approach generally have been vital concerns in those institutions seeking an organizational structure consistent with therapeutic patient care.

In response to the organizational handicaps of the past and in anticipation of fulfilling multiple future goals, an increasing number of mental hospitals have decentralized into separate units or sections, each of which autonomously provides a comprehensive array of services to the patients assigned to it. Under this plan, a single unit maintains administrative and clinical responsibility for the patient throughout his course of treatment and thereby seeks to reduce the depersonalized quality in staff-patient relationships created within large institutions. It is thought that Topeka State Hospital in 1951 was the first mental hospital to decentralize its services into a number of independent sections (Bay,

1964). During the following two decades, scores of public and V.A. psychiatric hospitals adopted similar structures so that a body of refined organizational propositions (Costonis, 1966) and experiential descriptions (Schulberg & Baker, 1969) has evolved around the unit plan as a strategy for institutional change. Hirschowitz (in press) has emphasized that a clear allocation of decisionmaking responsibility is essential, and he described four echelon levels with unique functions and decisions to be accomplished at each. The most basic level is the "firing line" which operates directly at the interface between hospital and consumer, while the topmost level is responsible for integrating the hospital's units and prospective guidance of the total enterprise. Despite a thriving literature, the transcripts of conferences sponsored a decade ago by the Mental Health Association of Southeastern Pennsylvania (1963) and the Milbank Memorial Fund (1964) continue to this day as basic primers for those interested in the decentralization of mental hospitals.

Goals of the Unit Plan

A variety of forces concerned with reorganizing psychiatric institutions has been attracted to the banner of the unit plan. Like many widely heralded salvations, unit plans have been inspired by diverse and sometimes incompatible goals which fall into three broad categories:

1. Improvement of a patient's care before, during, and subsequent to his hospitalization.
2. Modification of staff functions and training programs.
3. Expansion of the mental hospital into a comprehensive mental health center.

From the organizational perspective, the unit plan is generally considered to be vital for the hospital which wishes to expand its domain beyond inpatient services alone and to offer a comprehensive array of services. Through decentralization the hospital can reorganize itself to provide pre- and posthospital care as well as other services to the residents of a specific community while also developing appropriate linkages to the other community agencies. Increasing awareness of external environmental needs is evident in those hospitals which have unitized as components of community mental health programs, in contrast to the earlier changes which stemmed primarily from the pressures of an institution's internal difficulties. Another organizational goal sought through the unit plan is the equalization of available resources throughout the hospital instead of the traditionally higher staff-patient ratios on the intensive care unit. It also has been conjectured that the unit plan will reduce the hospital's average daily census and even permit it to calculate financial costs according to the specific utilization pattern of a given community.

The patient potentially benefits from the unit plan's goal of providing him with a specific group of staff who maintain continuous responsibility for him. Since patients cannot be transferred from one unit to another, more effective care results and the depersonalized ward atmosphere is reduced. In addition, the discharged patient can be helped to remain in the community when the same staff members maintain ongoing responsibility for his adjustment and continue to treat him as an outpatient.

The third category of goals to be achieved through the unit plan relates to efforts to modify staff functions and training programs. By decentralizing authority from the superintendent's and clinical director's offices to individual units, the locus of responsibility is shifted to a level at which many more staff members can feel constructively involved in patient care. Less stultifying and more creative roles can be developed when the degree of responsibility is commensurate with actual functions.

Although the unit plan is a potential administrative design which can simultaneously meet the goals of improved organizational efficiency, of improved patient care and of heightened staff creativity, there are numerous instances when the needs of these entities differ sufficiently to create considerable stress within the reorganized facility. Pepper (1964) has noted that the motivation of personnel supporting the unit plan includes the polarities of saving the hospital vs. destroying it. The hospital "savers" believe that this reorganization plan revitalizes the concept of the mental hospital as a viable entity and enables it to assume leadership in the care of the mentally ill. In contrast, the hospital "busters" think that the best strategy for doing away with the traditional mental hospital's sins is to decentralize and split it. The hospital ultimately will become so fragmented that it will be forced to integrate itself into the mainstream of the community's health and welfare network, a strategy which indeed is achieving results in the 1970s (Schulberg, 1972).

PATTERNS OF DECENTRALIZATION

Just as the goals of the unit plan have evolved and changed over the years, so have the organizational schemes for accomplishing these goals. Snow (1965) and Rowitz & Levy (1971) have described four different patterns, with the principle of decentralized authority for patient care a central and unwavering one in each pattern. It is evident that the manner in which at least three administrative problems are resolved consistently affects the ultimate organizational structure. Every hospital adopting a unit plan must decide upon the size of its autonomous units, the degree to which specialty functions and professional departments can be integrated within the decentralized units, and the manner in which newly admitted patients are to be distributed among the units.

The size of a decentralized unit is critical when the hospital's goals are those of increased patient-staff interaction and the reduction of chronicity. Many have proposed that units be kept at 100 beds so that little centralized hospitals with front wards and back wards do not recur, but this can create the need for an excessive number of personnel to staff so many independent units, especially if they have acute-patient wards. Another factor to be taken into account in determining unit size is that if the flow of patients between units is limited, the full utilization of bed capacity may be prevented in certain wards.

The second administrative issue requiring clarification is that of which specialty services and support facilities need to remain centralized and which can be integrated into the separate units. With the aim of avoiding back wards within the new units, many hospitals have not established distinctive reception services; acutely disturbed new admissions are treated on the same ward as chronic patients. The clinical feasibility of this arrangement seems clear in many instances, but others contend that poor morale is created among personnel when they are forced to care for acute, chronic and geriatric patients on the same ward.

A problem of increasing severity is the care of geriatric admissions, a difficulty often intensified by the mental hospital's failure to distinguish between those elderly patients who primarily need medical care and possibly could be treated elsewhere, in contrast to those whose needs are more psychiatric in nature. Also to be considered are the needs of a third geriatric group, i.e., the chronic schizophrenics who grow old and senile after many years of hospitalization. The administrative and clinical structure for treating the geriatric group varies considerably in unitized hospitals. Some have integrated elderly patients into every unit, but other institutions continue to maintain a centralized geriatric unit serving the entire hospital. Medicare funds are increasing the range of geriatric services available in the community, but optimal ways for utilizing the mental hospital in caring for the elderly are still unclear.

An equally urgent administrative dilemma in unitization is the manner in which to integrate existing professional departments and department heads into unit-based treatment teams. The multidisciplinary unit-focused team requires autonomy from departmental intervention if it is to be successful, and professional personnel inevitably are put in the position of having to choose between the conflicting role and loyalty expectations of their unit leader and department head. Some unitized hospitals have sought to minimize the professional staff tension by clearly restricting the role of department head to that of consultant. In some instances, in fact, staff conflict can only be resolved by completely abolishing the position of department head (Kiger, 1966).

The third administrative problem to be considered in selecting a decentralized organizational structure is the procedure for distributing newly admitted patients among the units. The changing way in which this issue is being resolved reflects the evolution of the mental hospital to a community mental health center, since it mirrors the facility's shift from an inpatient focus to a community orientation. Under the pioneering section plan established in the Kansas hospitals during the early 1950s, patients were randomly distributed among each of the sections. However, the Clarinda Plan (Garcia,

1960) and the second phase of the Kansas Plan (Jackson & Smith, 1961) called for each unit of the hospital to serve a specific geographic community and to accept all admissions from the area. These plans were precursors of the catchment-area concept now integral to the functioning of community mental health centers. We thus have moved in the past decade from acknowledging that "individual units could serve a specific geographic area [Brill et al., 1963]" to the prevailing opinion that units *should* be responsible for a designated community.

IMPLEMENTING THE UNIT PLAN AND CHANGING STAFF ROLES

Given the variety of organizational patterns and strategies for administering a decentralized program, how are they implemented and in what ways is this process facilitated or hindered by altered staff roles? It is widely recognized that procedures for implementing a unit plan must be considered within the context of modified staff functions since the changed role of the department head and other personnel is a major initial difficulty in the transition from a centralized to a decentralized facility. Consequently, a unit plan cannot be implemented by the superintendent's edict alone; he first must deal with complex personality and role factors.

The length and degree of preparation needed to implement a full unit plan differs among hospitals. Strong leadership by the superintendent is vital in reconciling divergent views, and his ability to reduce personnel insecurity ultimately will determine the success or failure of his plans. Wide variations in philosophy and planning can be seen between those institutions which decided to introduce a hospital-wide unit plan in one single step at a given point in time in contrast to those hospitals which considered it more judicious to proceed on a unit-by-unit basis over a longer period of time. Rowitz & Levy (1971) have described the movement from centralization to decentralization as usually passing through four phases during which the organizational structure, the formal communication network, the authority of service chiefs, the treatment orientation, etc., are progressively modified.

A key implementation problem is that of whether additional personnel are needed to operate a decentralized hospital. The superintendent cannot even begin to consider a unit plan if the hospital's staff is below a minimal level. The significant reduction of patient censuses in recent years has been instrumental in raising what were formerly skeletal staffs to more adequate ratios. Such initial reports as those by Brill et al. (1963) suggested that more personnel are required to run a subdivided hospital, even though the resulting benefits are beyond those achieved from increased personnel alone. Boyles & Waldrop (1967), however, found that a hospital with minimal staff can be unitized without increased personnel ratios and still produce beneficial outcomes.

As was noted previously, a frequent effect of the unit plan on staff roles is to remove department heads from line authority over the members of their discipline. If decentralization is to be implemented, department heads and clinical directors must relinquish supervisory authority over their personnel to the unit head and instead develop a guiding, consultative and training role with members of their discipline. Success in accomplishing this transition requires the paradoxical combination of leadership skills and ability to divest oneself of direct authority.

A beneficial effect of the unit plan on staff roles is that personnel can be freed from preconceived, rigidly defined functions and permitted to contribute to patient care to the best of their personal abilities. This evolution of mental health professionals toward generalized treatment team functions, particularly in community-based settings, runs counter to developments in other health fields faced with manpower shortages. In medicine, for example, specialties have proliferated so that optimal technical performance can be obtained in relation to organizational needs. These countertrends may stem from the fact that no specific theories about the etiology and treatment of mental illness have yet achieved widespread acceptance and, therefore, a generalist role is more appropriate for many mental health professionals.

Difficulty can arise, however, on those unit teams which pursue the generalist approach while the physician simultaneously retains ultimate responsibility and authority for the team's actions. Many physicians lack training and experience in supervisory skills, techniques of communication and delegation of authority and are ill-suited to the role of unit leader among generalist personnel. Thus, in acknowledging the overt benefits afforded many personnel by the generalist functions of the unit system, we shouldn't overlook the covert resentment which it also can engender among participating personnel. Babow & Johnson (1968) found that a positive attitude toward unitization is positively correlated with a sociotherapeutic orientation but negatively correlated with a somatotherapeutic orientation, authoritarianism and anomia.

Treatment Programs

Even more important than the effects of unitization upon the hospital's administrative structure and its personnel is the question of its impact upon patient treatment since this is a basic motivation for instituting the unit plan. The theoretical intent is that of moving from a hospital-oriented approach to a patient-centered one, and eliminating differential treatment patterns between the intensive and continued care services. Although some would contend that this benefit of the unit plan can be achieved without any significant modification of existing treatment techniques, the more common pattern is for therapeutic milieus to emerge as the new treatment of choice. Adherents of the therapeutic community are strong supporters of the unit system because it permits the same staff and patients to develop continuing interpersonal relationships and at many facilities this approach becomes the core of the treatment program. In fact, therapy groups can become so pervasive and overwhelming after unitization that the elderly segment of the hospital population was reported by Esquibel & Bower (1965) as finally pleading for an abeyance in staff enthusiasm for this approach. Zubowicz (1967) has experimented with patient-centered social systems which are established by subdividing all units into 15-patient-family groups which achieve, preserve and control societal values and standards of behavior. It has been conjectured that since units are organized according to the geographic communities which they serve, problems arising within the hospital's therapeutic community can be viewed as reflections of the environment from which patients come. No two hospital units need function alike, therefore, and each should develop a unique approach to its catchment area so that it can be attuned to the specific features of the community it serves.

A treatment problem of frequent concern under the unit system is that of how to deal with disturbed patients. Duran (1964) reported that in the pioneering work at

Clarinda Hospital, staff was able to eliminate special wards and seclusion facilities after unitization since the ward administrators, no longer allowed to transfer disturbed patients, developed treatment programs to which the patients responded. Similarly, the problems of housing male and female patients in the same building after unitization have been found to be minimal so that this traditional form of hospital segregation could also be eliminated. The general consensus which has emerged about the unit system is that it spontaneously gives rise to a variety of new clinical services since the staff feels that sanctions for meaningful functioning have been broadened considerably. Hospital personnel, for example, develop new intensive precare and aftercare services while also expanding traditional inpatient services (such as rehabilitation) into community clinics.

Accepting the significance of the unit plan as an administrative strategy for producing major change, we will now illustrate the previously discussed issues via a case study of Boston State Hospital's struggle to achieve appropriate decentralization. Between 1966 and the end of our study in 1969, the hospital lurched through a series of organizational changes which transformed its centralized, internally focused structure into one which could actively struggle with contemporary environmental pressures. Despite a series of administrative maneuvers which many staff members deemed chaotic and misdirected, in retrospect steady movement can be discerned toward a decentralized structure within which comprehensive clinical services are now provided to specific geographic catchment areas. As might be expected, these far-reaching changes were marked by intense struggles and resistances among competing forces with differing goals; generating conflicts similar to those initially described by Ishiyama & Grover (1960) in their study of a mental hospital where unitization was undertaken to reduce custodialism and increase therapy. The following case study, therefore, focuses upon the intertwined relationship of changing organizational goals and modified administrative and clinical structures, but particularly upon the mental hospital's transition from traditional concerns to community mental health emphases.

THE IMPETUS FOR CHANGE

Decentralization is motivated by varying needs and pressures which, when coalesced under a single banner, create a powerful impetus for change. The multiple goals sought by the diverse adherents of decentralization may or may not be compatible, however, at a given time. The potential for organizational conflict, therefore, is particularly rife during the transitional period as competing interests struggle to influence decisions for personal purposes. In analyzing the rationale for unitization at Boston State Hospital, it was evident that the institution's executives and staff were intent on solving problems in both the organization's administrative structure as well as in its clinical programs for patient care. Although these two categories of concern were complementary and interrelated, the pressure to resolve administrative and professional role conflicts often seemed paramount and consumed inordinate amounts of staff energy during the initial phases of decentralization. Consequently, improved patient-care services did not develop as rapidly and dramatically as some proponents of unitization had envisioned. To help understand these processes, we now will describe the administrative and patient-care pressures which motivated adoption of the initial unit plan in 1966.

Administrative Concerns

A centralized clinical, professional and business staff had guided Boston State Hospital's functioning for many years, but in 1965 several key staff members contended that a decentralized administrative structure would be more responsive to intraorganizational and community pressures for relevant services. Although this alternative structure had frequently been espoused during the previous decade, it had gained little support and remained a fanciful plan backed by few adherents. The balance of forces was shifting, however, and in 1965 many of the earlier obstacles to decentralization no longer seemed as formidable. Among the key developments permitting fresh consideration of the unit plan was the improved staff-patient ratio resulting from the hospital's reduced inpatient census. The managerial dilemma of how to spread an overly burdened staff among several comprehensive units no longer seemed insolvable. On the contrary, the superintendent was equally concerned with designing an administrative-clinical structure permitting growth opportunities for the bright, young professionals whom he had recently recruited to the hospital's staff.

The movement toward community-oriented activities creates unique complexities for the mental hospital groping for a decentralized structure. Boston State Hospital's inpatient census had been declining for several years, but the number of individuals being treated as outpatients had grown. A census conducted by the authors in October 1965 revealed that in addition to 1,880 inpatients, the institution also was caring for 1,200 individuals in various community-based subsystems; e.g., home treatment, aftercare, halfway house, foster care, outpatient clinic, etc. Although a proliferation of specialty subsystems maximized the potential for continuity of care, each subsystem in fact operated semiautonomously and thus paradoxically reduced organizational integration. The superintendent and other executives, therefore, deemed the unit plan's multiple managerial hierarchies more appropriate for the hospital's future administration since the unit system would provide a better span of control than the single centralized structure then governing the institution.

A related administrative problem in the unitization of evolving mental hospitals is that of staff ambiguity about the relative status of traditional institutional tasks and new community-based activities. At Boston State Hospital, the central reception service, with its psychoanalytic orientation, had long been the locus for prestigious inpatient clinical and training activities and, therefore, commanded a disproportionately large share of the institution's resources. The superintendent and others, however, wished to sanction the growth of innovative prestigious programs which would demonstrate a more social-psychiatric, community-focused orientation. The unit plan would diversify the reception service's resources and prestige, and create new power centers in units whose programs were more in keeping with the superintendent's goals.

Stable environments permit mental hospitals to plan with relative ease and to employ a primarily shortrange viewpoint in pondering the benefits of unitization. In complex, dynamic environments, however, planning requires a longer-range viewpoint since the organization must consider interacting with the community in ways which can only be dimly perceived (Baker, 1972). In the case of Boston State Hospital, the intraorganizational pressures for unitization were compounded by turbulent environmental developments. It seemed quite probable in 1966 that the state would enact a new Community Mental Health Law, among whose features would be the division of the city of Boston into several catchment areas with the hospital serving only one of them. Despite the centrality of the catchment-area concept to community mental health ideology and programs, the hospital's staff only dimly appreciated its profound relevance for their institution's future. Nevertheless, they recognized that the volume of inpatient admissions would be sharply curtailed after a period of time and that a broader variety of hospital programs would then be intensively focused upon a smaller geographic sector, rather than being thinly spread across the entire city. The shift to a decentralized organizational structure appeared compatible with the community-orientation in this new legislation.

Patient-Care Concerns

Although administrative pressures alone can be sufficiently critical to move adoption of the unit plan, concerns about patient care also contribute significantly to a hospital's decision to decentralize. Many clinicians who may be reluctant to support a reorganization which could strengthen the superintendent's quest for newly designed goals, become unit-plan adherents out of an awareness that patient care needs improvement.

Of greatest concern to the clinical staff at Boston State Hospital was the central reception service's increasing inability to screen and process the swelling number of individuals admitted for inpatient care. Admissions had grown to 1,500 by 1966, so that the overcrowded reception service was functioning primarily as a revolving door. A readmission rate of 50–60 percent was found among those discharged from the service, and increased staff, by itself, did not appear capable of resolving the problem. A more fruitful alternative appeared to be the creation of several new acute services among which inpatient admissions would be distributed. In tones reminiscent of what Pepper (1964) had characterized as hospital "busting," a senior psychiatrist maintained that the reception service's problems were insolvable within the existing structure. "It's too antiquated," he said. "You've got to wreck the machine and the unit plan is groundwork to do this."

Another prominent clinical problem in most mental hospitals is the discrepancy between the active efforts to treat acute patients and the meager treatment programs directed toward longterm patients. The imbalance has grown over the years because of selective personnel allocation policies and despite sporadic efforts to rectify this situation, there could be little doubt in the mid-1960s that most chronic patients received "back ward" care. At Boston State Hospital, the superintendent's emphasis upon rehabilitation services highlighted the problems of custodialism and lent further urgency to the search for an organizational scheme which would establish equitable staff-patient ratios throughout the institution. Decentralization through the unit plan was considered the solution.

Training Concerns

Organizations with multiple subsystems may find that changes in administrative structure and technological procedures are relatively more beneficial to some groupings than others, thus producing differing reactions to the transition. Mental hospitals with extensive educational subsystems have refined procedures for insuring centralized attention to training concerns, and the unit plan often is perceived by trainers as a threat to established procedures and priorities. At Boston State Hospital those responsible for psychiatric training recognized that under the unit structure, psychiatric residents would benefit from more evenly distributed patient loads and continuity of care would be enhanced. They feared, however, that with training occurring at the unit rather than at the central level, ideological and quality control over educational experiences would diminish. Analytically oriented educators were particularly concerned that some units would emphasize applied social-psychiatric concepts and techniques rather than meeting the resident's need for training in basic psychiatry, i.e., an understanding of intrapersonal dynamics and the techniques of psychotherapy. Thus, even though the hospital's clinical and administrative needs clearly justified adoption of the unit plan, decentralization was viewed with ambivalence from the training perspective since the new structure might generate more problems than benefits.

THE PHASES OF ADMINISTRATIVE TRANSITION

A crucial decision confronting those responsible for major organizational change is that of how much innovation the focal institution can constructively integrate within specified periods of time. Recognizing the overt anxiety and subtle resistances accompanying shifts from the status quo, the administrator must accurately gauge the resiliency and energy level of his staff and then move at a pace which rallies support rather than arousing defiance. In decentralizing a mental hospital, the superintendent must determine the rate at which departmental roles can be modified, clinical responsibilities shifted and patients transferred among various units. The patterns utilized to date have differed according to idiosyncratic institutional needs, and factors such as the superintendent's administrative style, organizational complexity, degree of staff support and scope of available resources.

As Boston State Hospital contemplated decentralization in late 1965, it was clear that magnitude and rate of change would be a crucial issue. Should all of the institution's many clinical and training programs be unitized in one fell swoop, or should the change proceed on a sequential basis over an extended period of time? The superintendent, whom many had perceived as seeking change for the sake of change, stated in late 1965 that total decentralization was too big an undertaking and "prudence, instinct and fear" led him to advocate a piecemeal approach. He preferred to start with a pilot comprehensive program on a unit which had already initiated social-psychiatric services, and to utilize the resulting experiences in decentralizing the remainder of the hospital. The director of the model pilot unit fully supported the strategy of limited implementation. Other senior staff were equally cognizant of unitization's complex systemic implications, but they feared that proceeding with only a model unit would detract from their own status and endanger resources already committed to their programs. They contended, therefore, that change must focus upon the total institution and not just a privileged section of it.

A paradoxical situation was thus created. The social psychiatrists who previously had been the organization's prime innovators now supported a cautious approach to unitization, while the more conservative, psychoanalytically oriented staff urged immediate and total decentralization of the entire hospital. Controversy between liberals and conservatives around the problem of change, thus, had shifted from ideological issues about patient care to concern for preserving existing domains, roles and resources. As a result, unitization was to be launched amid intense staff anxiety which delayed resolution of key systemic concerns; the initial pattern for decentralization was, therefore, to be repeatedly modified during the ensuing years.

UNITIZATION I

Institutions seeking improved organizational effectiveness through unitization often seek to defuse intense staff anxiety about change by initially adopting the subhospital model (Rowitz & Levy, 1971). This organizational pattern decentralizes certain clinical and administrative activities while continuing centralized control and responsibility for others. Although this model is fraught with complexities and inconsistencies, it reduces staff tension levels sufficiently for change processes to be activated.

Unitization I was undertaken at Boston State Hospital in the fall of 1966 within the general parameters of the subhospital model. A staff planning committee generated consensus for a framework whereby four new inpatient units, each accepting approximately 25 percent of the hospital's admissions, would function semiautonomously; existing specialty activities would retain centralized functions and controls. The plan, attuned more to the alleviation of staff anxieties than the comprehensive upgrading of clinical services, was based upon the following principles:

1. *Staff authority.* The new inpatient units would be semiautonomous and directed by a psychiatrist responsible for developing appropriate clinical programs. Personnel from several disciplines would work together as a team, and department heads would delegate responsibility for their professionals to the unit heads.

2. *Catchment area responsibilities*. Geographic catchment areas were to be assigned each unit, with the boundaries to be established by the new state Community Mental Health Act serving as a guide insofar as possible. Some gerrymandering would be necessary, however, so that equitable distribution of new admissions to all four units would be feasible.
3. *Continuity of care*. A central admissions unit would be retained in the interest of conserving manpower even though this would complicate the desired linkages and continuity of care between the community and its inpatient unit. Furthermore, the outpatient clinic would not be decentralized since the new plan was primarily concerned with inpatient services. The clinic director saw his program's function as that of providing psychotherapy for patients who could cope on their own and, therefore, opposed its inclusion in the hospital's revised inpatient unit structure.
4. *Specialty programs*. Clinical and research programs like the home treatment service and the adolescent unit were to continue intact because of their experimental nature and retain existing staffing patterns. Consequently, those inpatient units with specialty programs would benefit more than others despite the plan to deploy personnel on the basis of a unit's patient load. The training program for psychiatric residents, an activity with strong staff investment, would remain under the centralized direction of an analytically oriented training committee to counterbalance the anticipated impact of social psychiatric ward experiences. Residents would not be assigned to units which failed to meet established standards.

Irresolvable dilemmas about the tempo and magnitude

of organizational change become less complex once the rudiments of a plan achieve staff acceptance. The superintendent of Boston State Hospital, troubled with the choice of options which could either facilitate or retard systemic growth, concluded that adequate staff support existed for institutionwide change on the basis of the previously defined principles. The numerous steps required to implement Unitization I were completed uneventfully once the superintendent's decision was known; chronic patients were transferred to the former reception service, and acute clinical services were established on wards accustomed to treating only the chronically ill. The predominant staff feeling was one of relief that reorganization finally had been initiated, and a period of calm was sought by all so that the patient-centered purposes of unitization could now be pursued.

Approximately six months after the subhospital model was established, Babow & Johnson's (1968) questionnaire for measuring "Opinions on Unitization" was completed by 206 members of the hospital's professional staff. No differences in opinion were found on the seven-point scale among the personnel on different units, or among the members of the several professional disciplines. The general staff reaction to Unitization I (Table 6-1) was one of caution and uncertainty; most people were hesitant to associate changes in their own professional functions or in patient care with the new administrative structure.

Unitization I and Patient Care

Unitization I's effect upon patient care can be analyzed in a variety of ways. Utilizing the open system's model guiding our study of the changing mental hospital, we compared the input, throughput and output

Table 6–1
Opinions On Unitization

	Item	*Mean*	*S.D.*
**1.	Plans for unitization were carefully thought out in the hospital.	4.94	1.80
*2.	During the period of establishing unitization, fewer patients have improved and more have become worse.	5.26	1.46
**3.	Unitization has increased the efficiency of communication in the hospital.	4.25	2.00
*4.	Unitization has stirred up jealousies and resentments in the treatment team.	4.23	1.89
*5.	This hospital was unitized because unitization is currently the popular way of thinking.	3.60	1.91
*6.	Under unitization, more friction has resulted from team members being supervised by people in other fields as well as by people in their own field.	4.47	1.74
**7.	Unitization has led to improved patient care in the hospital.	5.18	1.68
**8.	For me, there has been considerable change since unitization.	4.35	2.04
*9.	With unitization, some departments are losing their sense of identity and autonomy in the emphasis on the medically run treatment team.	4.03	1.79
**10.	Unitization has reduced rivalries and frictions within the treatment team.	3.65	1.69
**11.	Unitization has had a positive effect on staff morale.	4.41	1.76
*12.	I don't like unitization.	5.53	1.69

* Strongly agree = 1; strongly disagree = 7
** Strongly disagree = 1; strongly agree = 7

measures for a cohort of inpatient admissions prior and subsequent to this administrative restructuring. Within our conceptual framework it was relevant to consider unitization's impact upon: (1) the nature of inpatient admissions from a specific geographic area; (2) the hospital's treatment services for these individuals; and (3) the hospital's ability to discharge these persons from the institution. This analysis was conducted by comparing the characteristics, treatment and disposition of a pre–Unitization I cohort with those of a post–Unitization I cohort. The former group consisted of 100 randomly selected persons admitted to Boston State Hospital from the Dorchester neighborhoods of its catchment area between January 1 and June 30, 1965; the latter group consisted of all 218 inpatient admissions from the same geographic area between January 1 and June 30, 1967.

A human service organization's ability to generate acceptable outputs is very much related to the characteristics of the individuals for whom it accepts responsibility. The patient inputs to Boston State Hospital were changing at the time of Unitization I's launching in the fall of 1966 as the result of ethnic shifts in the surrounding community. For example, the percentage of blacks among Dorchester inpatient admissions rose from 10 percent to 15 percent of the total between 1965 and 1967. Change was also evident in the two cohorts' age-distribution. The percentage between 25 and 59 years of age increased from 51 percent to 63 percent of the total between 1965 and 1967; the proportion below 25 and over 60 dropped. On other personal traits, however, the pre- and post-unitization cohorts were similar. Both in 1965 and 1967 the sex distribution was 45 percent male, 55 percent female; religious preference was 60 percent Catholic, 20 percent Protestant and 17 percent Jewish; and approximately 65 percent were not living with a spouse.

In terms of clinical characteristics, we found that al-

Table 6-2
Previous Hospitalization of
Pre- and Post-Unitization I Admission Cohorts

Facility	1965 *No. & %*	1967 *No.*	*%*
No information, unknown	8	14	6
BSH alone	10	39	18
BSH and other hospitals	27	71	33
Other psychiatric hospitals	14	27	12
General medical hospitals	26	15	7
No previous hospitalization	15	52	24
	100	218	100

though the admission diagnoses for the two cohorts were similar, their histories of previous psychiatric care were indeed different (Table 6-2). Only 7 percent of the post–Unitization I cohort had first been hospitalized in general medical facilities, in contrast to 26 percent of the pre–Unitization I group which had been treated earlier in such hospitals. Conversely, 51 percent of the 1967 cohort as against only 37 percent of the 1965 group was known to Boston State Hospital staff from previous admissions to their institution. Furthermore, the 1967 group contained a larger proportion of individuals for whom this admission was the initial one than was the case for the 1965 group. Thus, the post-Unitization I cohort simultaneously was more chronic and more acute in relation to its history of care at Boston State Hospital. This may have resulted from the community and staff's growing perception of the institution as an open one providing continuity of care; the percentage of voluntary inpatient admissions rose from 7 percent to 17 percent between 1965 and 1967, indicating a growing comfort among both patients and professionals about facilitating entry to and exit from the hospital.

As in most institutions, Unitization I was undertaken at Boston State Hospital in 1966 to achieve a variety of goals. Primary among the patient-oriented ones was the improving of throughput processes—i.e., treatment services—for the inpatients whom the hospital hoped to discharge back into the community. Improved clinical service includes better continuity of care, more individualized therapy, a greater range of treatment options, etc. We, therefore, reviewed available hospital records to determine whether treatment patterns for the pre- and postunitization cohorts differed on any of such measures.

Inpatient continuity of care may be operationally defined in terms of the number of wards on which a patient is treated during the course of a hospitalization. The fewer the wards, the more continuous is treatment. We found that in both 1965 and 1967 two-thirds of all new admissions were treated on but a single ward, another 24 percent were treated on two wards, and 11 percent on three wards or more. Thus, degree of continuity in inpatient care was not altered by unitization.

A second criterion of improved treatment services is whether the hospital is providing specific therapy to its patients. A 1965 survey of the hospital's clinical patterns had revealed a growing number of patients on drug regimens and in verbal therapies (Schulberg, Notman, & Bookin, 1967). Since patient records contained better data about the former than the latter treatment, we reviewed the records to ascertain the impact of 1966's unitization upon drug administration. Table 6-3 indicates that the postunitization cohort received more drugs than did the preunitization group at either time of hospitalization, during hospitalization, or at point of discharge. The increased use of medications was particularly sharp in regard to the major tranquilizers; 70 percent more patients received such prescriptions in 1967 than in 1965. The hospital's earlier trend towards increased use

Table 6-3
Percentage of Patients Receiving Medication During Hospitalization

Type of Drug	*Year* 1965	1967
Major tranquilizers	37%	63%
Minor tranquilizers	18%	26%
Anti-depressants	19%	22%
Side-effects	8%	19%
Sleeping medication	51%	64%
Non-psychotropic	38%	52%

of drugs was thus seen to be continuing, if not accelerating, subsequent to unitization.

Finally, in analyzing a hospital's treatment strategies, it is relevant to inquire about the flexibility with which a patient's management is determined. For example, are all admitted persons maintained on 24-hour inpatient status, or are some treated through day and night hospital arrangements? A review of hospital records for our pre- and postunitization cohorts revealed that the percentage of patients participating in day care during the hospitalization episode under study rose from 6 percent in 1965 to 15 percent in 1967. Thus, growing clinical flexibility in meeting patient needs, as measured by this parameter, was evident subsequent to Unitization I.

This analysis of the hospital's ability to improve treatment procedures through unitization is necessarily sketchy because of records limitations, but greater efforts were discerned to involve more patients in specific therapeutic care. Drug prescriptions continued to increase, and the role and significance of this inpatient treatment will be discussed more fully in Chapter 10. An increased number of inpatients participated in day care subsequent to this restructuring. On the other hand, continuity of care by minimizing ward transfers was not altered by unitization.

The purpose of comparing an organization's throughput processes at different points in time is to determine whether any intervening administrative or technological modifications have affected its outputs. Does the administrative process of unitizing a mental hospital improve the organization's subsequent ability to rapidly and effectively discharge a cohort of new admissions back to the community? More specifically, does the outcome of hospitalization improve, is the length of initial hospitalization shortened, is discharge planning refined, and is the total annual duration of hospital stay curtailed?

The impact of Unitization I upon the cohort of Dorchester residents admitted to Boston State Hospital in 1967 was studied through a comparison of its outcome within 12 months of initial hospitalization with that for the 1965 cohort. Interestingly enough, the length of initial hospital stay increased from a median of 17.5 days in 1965 to 28 days in 1967, a clinical course counter to the national trend of shortened inpatient care. At Boston State Hospital, however, unitization was explicitly intended to curtail the nontherapeutic, revolving-door services of its overcrowded admissions unit; after the restructuring, patients were indeed discharged less rapidly.

Did the lengthened inpatient stay improve the hospital staff's ability to plan specific postdischarge aftercare for released inpatients? Since such planning is a key determinant of a patient's readjustment to community living, we searched clinical records for such information. Some improvement was found in the specificity of discharge planning after unitization. Only 39 percent of the 1965 cohort was to be followed-up at Boston State Hospital or elsewhere, while such plans were made for 46 percent of the 1967 cohort.

When the basic outcome of hospitalization for the 1965 and 1967 cohorts was compared, no change was

Table 6-4
Outcome of Inpatient Admission

Outcome	1965 *No. & %*	1967 *No.*	*%*
Died in hospital	5	9	4
Still in hospital	8	20	9
Discharged within 12 months	87	189	87
	100	218	100

found (Table 6-4). Of the total groups, 87 percent were discharged within 12 months of admission, 8 percent remained hospitalized and 5 percent died as inpatients at both time periods. However, the hospital's intent to further the goal of reintegrating discharged patients back within their community through unitization did affect the destination of those released from the institution. We found that 56 percent of the 1967 group versus only 50 percent of the 1965 group returned to their own or relatives' homes. Only 17 percent of the 1967 cohort was transferred from Boston State Hospital to other residential facilities such as nursing homes and hospitals, in contrast to 31 percent of the 1965 cohort which left the mental hospital for such alternative facilities.

The "quality" of the hospital's output of treated patients can also be assessed in terms of the success with which these people remain out of the institution subsequent to discharge. A check of hospital records for those members of the 1965 and 1967 cohorts discharged within 12 months of admission revealed that the rehospitalization rate within this yearlong timespan jumped from 17 percent for the preunitization cohort to 29 percent for the postunitization cohort. The median number of days between discharge and readmission dropped from

114 for the 1965 group to 96 for the 1967 group. As a correlate of this decrease, the median number of days spent by the 1967 cohort as inpatients at Boston State Hospital during the 12 months subsequent to focal admission rose to 42 from the median of 27 for the 1965 cohort.

In summary, our comparison of the hospital's outputs subsequent to Unitization I with those evident prior to this administrative change revealed that at the latter point in time: (1) discharges were less precipitous, (2) aftercare was somewhat better planned and (3) growing numbers of patients returned to community residences. On the other hand, we also found that for the postunitization cohort: (4) readmission rates had increased, (5) patients were returning more rapidly to the hospital and (6) patients were spending more days of the year as hospital residents. These research findings suggested that while Unitization I had generated some improvements in clinical care, significant shortcomings still remained. Indeed, the hospital's staff itself quickly recognized that the initial restructuring of their organization's clinical subsystems was but a start and that more far-reaching changes would be needed in the near future if lingering difficulties were to be dispelled.

UNITIZATION II

When a mental hospital's staff is sufficiently motivated to implement even rudimentary unitization, the subhospital model is adequate for activating change processes. The model is less than optimal over protracted periods of time, however, since it leaves unresolved the issue of centralized versus decentralized functions and responsibilities, and it obfuscates the processes for designing organizational priorities and programs. The subhospital model's negative features became evident at Boston State Hospital within a year of implementing Unitization I. Each new inpatient unit increasingly was providing autonomous services and screening its own admissions during weekdays, but during evenings and weekends the hospital reverted to its former structure and functioned in a centralized rather than decentralized fashion. Consequently, a tranquil period of organizational growth emphasizing improved patient care failed to develop, and tension and uncertainty again engulfed the hospital staff responsible for programmatic success. Unit leaders and hospital executives expressed dissatisfaction with the organization's administrative structure, personnel deployment, and standards of patient care. The following issues were of specific concern:

1. *Degree of decentralized authority*. The unit system is intended to provide decentralized services with greater independence in developing appropriate programs. The central administration must also retain institutionwide authority and standard setting prerogatives, however, lest the organization lose its identity and devolve into a series of fragmented subsystems. Boston State Hospital had not determined an appropriate balance between centralized and decentralized authority needs and, furthermore, interunit relationships remained ambiguous. Could the units directly negotiate programs and exchange resources with each other, or must such transactions be channeled through the central administration?
2. *Parity among units*. Adherents of orderly organizational growth contend that equalization of patient load and staff resources must be achieved among the decentralized units, preferably within the guidelines of a master plan. If any unit remains overly large and understaffed, patient care will

not improve. Although the principle of parity based upon a master plan appealed to many at Boston State Hospital, the principle's implementation proceeded haltingly. The guiding master plan, based upon the subhospital model of both centralized and decentralized structures, did not insure parity since it maintained specialty staffing arrangements. Additionally, the superintendent's penchant for stimulating interunit competition and encouraging experimental ventures on whatever units he deemed appropriate further obfuscated the administration's commitment to parity among units.

3. *Continuity of care.* Although the community mental health goal of continuity of care often is furthered by the unit plan, this goal was not being adequately addressed at Boston State Hospital. Prehospitalization and aftercare programs continued to function independently of the newly decentralized inpatient units, with linkages of an only tenuous nature. To be sure, the subhospital model's tolerance for fragmented services had simplified the unit system's introduction. Continuation of this fragmented pattern seemed arbitrary and anachronistic, however, at a time when the goal of continuity of care was receiving increased priority. The superintendent's designation of the well-established home treatment service, the hospital's initial venture into community psychiatry, as an "experimental program" requiring independence from the new units, particularly incensed those espousing formal integration of outpatient and inpatient services.

4. *Acute and chronic patients.* The state's new Community Mental Health Act had defined the mental hospital's role as that of providing comprehensive

care to the residents of its own catchment area, and only longterm care to the residents of neighboring catchment areas. As the differential level of organizational commitment and resource investment implied by the act became clear, the hospital staff wondered about the wisdom of having recently established four intensive inpatient units. Perhaps it would be more efficient to consolidate scarce resources for the care of acute admissions from the hospital's own catchment area in a single unit, while utilizing proportionately fewer of the institution's remaining personnel and facilities to provide the longterm care required by chronic patients who reside in Boston's other catchment areas.

These four concerns highlighted the administrative and programmatic limitations of Unitization I, and the institution's staff realized that the subhospital model would require modification. The problem was that of how simultaneously to accommodate the contradictory thrusts towards decentralized authority and parity among units, while maintaining centralized systemic unity so that continuity of care would be enhanced and planning for new organizational purposes would be furthered. The lack of a longterm master plan geared both to internal pressures and rapidly changing environmental demands was sorely felt.

Even after decentralization has been initiated, the mental hospital's superintendent continues to play a key leadership role in resolving organizational dilemmas. Dr. Greenblatt resigned in June 1967 as superintendent of Boston State Hospital to become the commissioner of his state's department of mental health, and a leadership vacuum was created by his departure. The new superintendent, Dr. Jonathan Cole, keenly supported the hospital's social-psychiatric orientation, but, like many new executives, preferred to learn about the hospital's programs and personnel before resolving Unitization I's lingering complexities. A respite was thus provided to those intent on maintaining the initial pattern, but a sense of inevitable further change loomed heavily on the organization's horizon.

Once having launched upon the path of decentralization, the community-oriented mental hospital can best unravel emerging problems within guidelines attuned to both environmental changes as well as intraorganizational concerns. Within a year after becoming superintendent, Dr. Cole concluded that his hospital's future role would primarily be that of providing community mental health services to but one of Boston's several catchment areas—a role best fulfilled by consolidating two of the new inpatient units into a single comprehensive one. The consolidated unit would emphasize short-term hospitalization for new admissions and intensive rehabilitation for longterm patients. Sheltered community living arrangements would be established and visited by mobile aftercare teams. The two remaining inpatient units established in Unitization I would no longer accept acute admissions; instead they would serve as backup facilities for the mental health centers in neighboring catchment areas.

The organizational pattern suggested by the superintendent for Unitization II approximates what Rowitz & Levy (1971) have termed the "decentralized transitional" model. This phase of change tends to be highly active; charged emotions are rampant, and ambivalence about decentralization once again pervades the organization. Since the superintendent's decision to emphasize services for the hospital's own catchment area would affect resource deployment, latent resistances to unitization and fears about the loss of authority once again surfaced at all staff levels. As a compromise, it was agreed to maintain the outpatient clinic, the home treatment service and other specialized programs as independent of the inpatient unit despite the impediments thus caused to continuity of care. The decentralized transitional model of Unitization II was quickly implemented, and it symbolized a growing organizational priority for comprehensive catchment-area services. Thus, decentralized inpatient resources had now been regrouped to further this commitment, but the anachronistically fragmented community-based programs would still require administrative restructuring if the aim of continuity of care was to be fully achieved.

UNITIZATION III

Mental hospitals which decentralize their administrative and clinical structures do so to insure more effective management and to improve patient care. Neither goal can be achieved until staff anxieties are placated, a process whose duration is related to administrative style, organizational complexity, stability of a master plan, etc. At Boston State Hospital, staff preoccupation with personal domains and changing roles extended over a period of several years because of: (a) senior staff ambivalence toward dealing with administrative matters; (b) greater staff skill in dealing with individual patients than with organizational dynamics; (c) the superintendents' philosophy of encouraging senior staff to develop personal interests even though these efforts ultimately might not comprise a total institutional program; and (d) the fluctuating nature of environmental developments which subjected the hospital to unexpected program shifts.

By 1969, the hospital's planning increasingly centered upon its role as a community mental health center, but widely divergent opinions continued to be expressed about these two key dimensions.

1. *Institutional versus community focus.* Should the hospital's future structure reflect such existing constraints as the large backlog of chronic patients and limited physical facilities, or should it be geared towards an optimal model of community mental health services? The institutionally focused approach would emphasize improved inpatient services, particularly for the chronic patient, while the ideal model would deemphasize inpatient care and design programs geared to the needs of the geographic sectors comprising the hospital's own catchment area.
2. *Specialist versus generalist staff functions.* Should staff teams continue to be organized according to specialist clinical functions, such as inpatient and outpatient care; or should staff be reorganized as generalists so that each team provides comprehensive services to delimited neighborhoods? The specialist teams would capitalize on the unique skills of different personnel, while the generalist teams could more easily insure continuity of care for all patients from their geographic areas.

In analyzing the hospital's movement toward a community mental health orientation, it was evident by 1969 that the staff was providing all ten of the federally defined essential and desirable clinical services comprising a comprehensive program. Yet, only the most biased observer would contend that the hospital truly had become an effective community mental health center. No framework existed as yet for coalescing all of the service components into a total system. The superintendent's office constituted the only nexus within which the program strands could be linked, an arrangement strikingly similar to the unsatisfactory administrative structure which existed prior to the initial unitization in 1966. The superintendent had hoped that collaborative arrangements would be devised by the directors of the inpatient, outpatient and home treatment units serving the hospital's catchment area, but this voluntary collaboration had not yet occurred. Therefore, a new decentralization strategy was required.

Consideration of the options available for Unitization III led the administration to conclude that community mental health services to the hospital's catchment area are best structured around geographic parameters rather than clinical specialties. The existing inpatient, outpatient, home treatment and primary prevention units would be integrated and then decentralized into three new comprehensive units, each with staff functioning as generalists and responsible for total services to a sector of the hospital's catchment area. This pattern would finally decentralize the institution and permit interdisciplinary teams to insure continuity of care, eliminating the difficulties incurred in moving patients from one level of clinical care to the next.

The authors' active study of the hospital's development terminated at this key point in its history. Continuing contacts have made us aware, however, that geographically focused comprehensive units have emerged as the organizational vehicle for delivering clinical services to the assigned catchment area. Thus, approximately five years passed from the introduction of Unitization I, whose decentralized services were restricted to an inpatient focus and primarily suited staff needs, to the completion of Unitization III, which has strived to decentralize administrative and clinical structures within the parameters of community mental health principles. More recent organizational activities have focused upon the coordination of hospital programs with those of community agencies. Thus, for the first time in its history, the hospital is functioning more as an environmentally oriented, open system rather than an internally preoccupied, closed system.

LINKS TO LOCAL MENTAL HEALTH CENTERS

Program planners at the statewide and federal levels anticipated in the mid-1960s that newly established community mental health centers (CMHC's) would replace mental hospitals. Despite this initial expectation, it quickly became evident that mental hospitals would have to continue fulfilling various clinical purposes, including inpatient treatment for CMHC patients when local facilities are lacking, and the caring for long-term patients transferred from CMHC's. Planners hoped that such programs would be jointly operated by the mental hospital and the CMHC through specific administrative arrangements best suited to local conditions. For example, a mental hospital could designate certain of its units as affiliates of neighboring CMHC's, thereby facilitating patient transfers and staff communications. The neighboring CMHC's, in turn, could assume partial or full responsibility for their affiliated units at the mental hospital, a particularly feasible arrangement when travel time from one facility to the other is less than 45 minutes. Given the exigencies of program needs in many localities, the contemporary mental hospital thus has been presented a dual mandate: (1) to decentralize anachronistic clinical subsystems so as to provide integrated comprehensive services to its own catchment area; and (2) to establish decentralized units with effective linkages to neighboring CMHC's. The earlier sections of this chapter have reviewed strategies for meeting the first function, and we now will consider the issues pertaining to the second.

In contrast to the growing clarity with which mental hospitals have learned to unitize for purposes of delivering community-oriented services, considerable confusion and even outright opposition beclouds the development of linkages between mental hospitals and CMHC's. This is not surprising since interorganizational relationships are affected by such complex variables as allocation of resources, administrative auspices and domain concerns. A national study by the authors in 1971 of relationships between mental hospitals and CMHC's found that only minimal cooperation and staff exchanges occur between these two types of psychiatric facilities. Maximum interaction occurred when both the mental hospital and the CMHC operate under public auspices, a formal affiliation agreement exists between them, and the facilities are less than 45 minutes traveling time from each other.

The Massachusetts Community Mental Health Act mandated Boston State Hospital to provide longterm care and other special services to the residents of its neighboring catchment areas. The hospital's superintendent and staff, therefore, undertook negotiations in late 1966 with the executives of nearby mental health centers to determine mutually relevant clinical services and clarify procedures for resource exchange. Whether the parties agree to a formal affiliative arrangement significantly affects the nature of subsequent interorganizational linkages. We, consequently, will distinguish mental hospital–CMHC relationships based upon a contractual agreement from those linkages established upon a noncontractual basis.

Contractual Linkages

Soon after Boston State Hospital undertook Unitization I in 1966, the medical school operating a neighboring community mental health program proposed a formal contract whereby it would partially staff the hospital inpatient unit serving residents of its catchment area. The interorganizational agreement clearly could be mutually beneficial. An affiliated unit was vital to the medical school's quest for federal community mental health center staffing funds, while the hospital would gain additional personnel to operate the inpatient unit already serving patients from the medical school's catchment area. However, having functioned for decades as a closed system with little resource exchange, the contract's unprecedented provisions raised such dilemmas as the following for the hospital:

1. Would the affiliated unit be closely associated with, or independent of other hospital programs? For example, would the medical school's psychiatric residents assigned to the affiliated unit participate in the medical school's or the hospital's training program, or both?
2. Would the affiliated unit's director be on the staff of and responsible to the medical school, the hospital or both?
3. How many and what types of personnel would the medical school assign from its staffing grant to the hospital's inpatient facility? Who would be responsible for recruiting and supervising these personnel?

The hospital's initial stand on these issues was indecisive since: (a) Unitization I, with its inherent ambiguities, had been but recently undertaken; (b) the hospital had not set a priority for new community mental health functions directed toward its own catchment area in relation to continuing institutional services for the larger region; and (c) staff was uncomfortable in loosening organizational boundaries to the extent required by the affiliative agreement. Nevertheless, when the medical school obtained a federal staffing grant in 1968, an affiliated unit was established with programs featuring a high degree of patient and staff exchange.

The medical school's "continuity team," whose functions are similar to those of the expediters trained by Hansell et al. (1968), has helped foster continuity of care since it is responsible for providing the links between precare, inpatient and aftercare services, thus insuring that each patient's movement through the relevant elements of the total community mental health system is maximally coordinated. Continuity of care has been particularly facilitated for medical school catchment-area patients since they are admitted directly to the affiliated inpatient unit and need not be processed through the hospital's central admitting service. On the other hand, geriatric patients and those individuals requiring medical attention are treated elsewhere within the hospital and not on the affiliated unit.

As the programs of an affiliated unit develop and expand, uncertainty about the unit's identity and primary organizational affiliation inevitably generates conflicting loyalties among staff. The administrators of the sponsoring organizations also hesitate to assign the unit a high priority in resource allocation. Discussions between Boston State Hospital and the medical school revealed that although the affiliated unit had refined features worthy of emulation elsewhere, there were also many persistent problems. Administrative controls were ambiguous, the affiliated unit's physical facilities at the hospital were inadequate, staffing patterns vacillated, etc. As the authors completed their research at the hospital in 1969, the medical school was seeking to shift its affiliated unit to a nearby general hospital. Thus, even when an interorganizational agreement is of initially mutual benefit, changing program needs and competing organizational priorities require that the mental hospital and the community mental health center constantly review the contract's provisions if it is to remain viable and effective.

Noncontractual Linkages

In contrast with the intensive, albeit fluctuating relations which mental hospitals develop with contractually affiliated community mental health centers, noncontractual program linkages are vaguer, if not absent. A delicate equilibrium exists between the admissions policies, treatment services, training programs and resource allocations of the concerned institutions, and in the absence of pressure to affiliate, each participant exercises considerable caution in negotiating linkages for continuity of patient care. From the perspective of the mental hospital, the following issues are of concern as it ponders whether to provide specialized facilities for neighboring mental health centers:

1. Given a relative dearth of personnel, assigning hospital staff to treatment programs for the patients of neighboring centers detracts from the institution's ability to expand community mental health services for its own catchment area. Nevertheless, systemic considerations require that the hospital provide both local and regional services.
2. If the mental hospital readily accepts all patients transferred from neighboring centers, it can become a "dumping ground" for difficult or undesirable cases. How can the institution restrict its services to those selected individuals capable of benefiting from its limited resources?
3. How can positive morale be maintained among the hospital personnel staffing wards with patients transferred from neighboring centers? The

personnel's status is ambiguous since the hospital emphasizes the upgrading of its own catchment-area units, while the centers view backup hospital units as marginal appendages.

4. Can neighboring mental health centers be induced to accept responsibility for all chronic patients discharged from the hospital into their catchment area, or will the centers restrict aftercare services to those patients initially referred by them to the mental hospital?

The efforts made by Boston State Hospital and several neighboring mental health centers, as well as attempts by similar organizations elsewhere in the country, to design interorganizational linkages can be viewed as a frustrating flirtation. The concerned parties recognize the need for cooperative arrangements and yet exercise profound ambivalence in resolving troublesome issues. For example, the neighboring mental health centers may be dissatisfied with the physical facilities and clinical services available to their catchment-area patients at the mental hospital, but are unwilling to commit the major resources needed to rectify the situation. The hospital, on the other hand, is crystallizing its role as a comprehensive center for its own catchment area and, consequently, assigns minimal attention and resources to the treatment of patients from other parts of the city, viewing continued treatment and special services for noncatchment-area residents as a drain upon limited personnel and physical facilities. An increasingly firm stance has been assumed by some mental hospitals in negotiating any joint program which possibly could detract from plans for the hospital's own catchment area. For example, in a December 1970 memo to the Commissioner of the Massachusetts Department of Mental Health, Boston State Hospital's assistant superintendent noted that the nature of regional backup programs still required thoughtful, longrange planning and that it is questionable whether the mental hospital should operate continued treatment and special services wards for the neighboring mental health centers. Thus, in the absence of contractual agreements for affiliated units, mental hospitals and community mental health centers founder upon a host of obstacles in designing interorganizational linkages. Many clinical and administrative issues remain to be answered as the mental hospital confronts the formidable task of structuring its resources to meet the mandated function of providing continuing care and selected services to the residents of neighboring catchment areas.

The Impact of Unitization

The opportunity to radically redesign an organization with changing purposes is relatively rare, and most administrators must be content to modify existing structures through transitional procedures. This chapter has analyzed the tortuous path followed by a mental hospital in decentralizing its administrative and clinical structures so as to fulfill the contemporary functions mandated for it by the state Community Mental Health Act. The processes observed at Boston State Hospital highlight the fact that smoothness of transition is affected by the organization's ability to undertake longterm planning, and to choose appropriate change strategies. A clear conception of the ultimate goal and active staff participation in the planning engender support, while oscillation and secretiveness usually provoke wrath and resistance. Unitization is also abetted and constrained by such complex forces as the personalities of key staff members, differing theoretical orientations, limited physical facilities, fluctuating program mandates from the state and federal governments and shifting demands for inpatient and outpatient care. Despite the interwoven nature of these diverse factors, many observers are impressed by the powerful manner in which the personal concerns of staff members and their jurisdictional struggles dominate and preempt program choices. For example, unitization at Boston State Hospital remained a weekday phenomenon for several years because of key staff's unwillingness to be on duty evenings and weekends. It must also be emphasized, however, that executive policymaking style can reinforce staff preoccupation with personal roles. If new program directions are undertaken with but tenuous commitments, ensuing rumors of change can lead staff to fear capricious administrative actions.

The evaluation of health programs is generally fraught with conceptual and methodological complexities and the same is true in assessing the mental hospital unit plan, particularly because of the diverse goals which it is designed to simultaneously fulfill. When the unit plan's impact is evaluated from the objective, statistical viewpoint, the most striking and recurring finding is that many decentralized hospitals successfully reduce their inpatient populations by approximately 50 percent within a period of three to five years (Duran, 1964; Kiger, 1966), a rate far exceeding that of most traditionally organized facilities. Convincing evidence in this regard can be seen in Smith et al.'s (1965) finding that even though drugs had been used for five years at Colorado State Hospital, no significant population decrement occurred until after the abrupt administrative and organizational changes induced by unitization. More recently, Ellsworth et al. (1972) studied 39 V.A. psychiatric hospitals with unit systems. They found that the most productive institutions, as measured by an increase in turnover rates and a decrease in longterm residents, had special placement programs, smaller treatment units and competition between unit staffs.

When the unit plan's impact is considered from the subjective viewpoint of those who have participated in the decentralization and subsequent operation of large mental hospitals, this approach generally is thought to be beneficial and worth replicating elsewhere. In fact, its adherents develop a fervent, cultist ardor intended to produce a bandwagon movement toward the unit plan in all of the country's mental hospitals. Supporters assert that trimmer tables of organization result when psychiatric functions are distinguished and managed within the unit structure. In addition to the various benefits cited earlier in this chapter, the unit plan furthers comprehensive programs for the hospital's catchment-area residents and insures better continuity of patient care. From another perspective, however, decentralization creates negative side-effects. Organizational integrity may be diminished and priorities obscured as the transitional phases of unitization transform the institution into a collection of little hospitals, making it exceedingly difficult to assess the systemic implications of every new proposed program thrust.

Nevertheless, in an era when community mental health principles increasingly guide the mental hospital's functions, the unit plan is vital for the design of clinical programs incorporating contemporary rationales and purposes. Decentralization permits program emphasis to shift from a preoccupation with inpatient services toward a greater concern for patient care prior and subsequent to hospitalization. The real and imagined distinctions between treating a patient in the hospital and in his community are dissolved as unit staff and community caregivers gain greater comfort in working with each other. To be sure, the unit plan's stimulation of community mental health–oriented services has been slow and deliberate, reflecting at least partially the hospital staff's lingering ambiguity about program purposes. Some mental hospital personnel are willing to expand the institution's functions beyond narrowly defined clinical responsibilities and to grapple with those aspects of community life adversely affecting an individual's mental health. However, most staff members deem it inappropriate for their individual units to undertake social reform and, thus, they have emphasized clinically oriented activities in community settings. Within this framework of responsibility, the unit structure has undoubtedly permitted the flow and exchange of patients between hospital and community in a much smoother manner.

Finally, it should be noted that although unitization has lent clarity to the design of comprehensive services for the mental hospital's catchment area, the optimal structure for organizing the hospital's backup services so as to meet the needs of neighboring mental health centers still remains elusive. The administrative complexities in designing workable interorganizational links have been formidable, and the negotiations continue to be focused upon personnel exchanges and supervisory controls rather than strategies of patient treatment. Almost a decade ago, Bay (1964) warned that there is no logical reason to assume that unitization will serve all of the mental hospital's diverse needs. Time has justified his reservations. Ellsworth et al. (1972) reported that despite favorable staff reaction and increased hospital productivity under the unit system, V.A. hospitals are again moving toward more specialized treatment wards. We would suggest that there now is no single permanent solution to the mental hospital's organizational dilemmas. Its program mandates fluctuate with vacillating societal values and changing ideologically tinged technologies. Perhaps an ultimate breakthrough into the causes and treatment of mental illness will promote administrative and clinical structures based on facts rather than fads.

7. *Staff Ideology at a Mental Hospital*

A review of mental health program development during the past century reveals a succession of ideological movements, each of which produced unique constellations of theory and technology. Although serving as powerful determinants of program directions while in vogue, each of the movements has fallen into disrepute in the face of changing societal influences. In Chapter 3 we described the characteristics of community mental health ideology and its predominant influence on the nature of mental health undertakings during the 1960s. Among the ideology's fundamental purposes is the merging of traditional humanistic values with contemporary service arrangements so as to better meet patients' needs. The ideology's conceptual beliefs include the following five themes: a population focus, primary prevention, social treatment goals, comprehensive continuity of care and total community involvement.

The community mental health movement grew rapidly and extensively in its influence upon mental health workers, but the movement's ideology has by no means met with uniform acceptance among all of the various mental health professions. In the study which originally developed the Community Mental Health Ideology Scale (Baker & Schulberg, 1967), significant differences in degree and type of commitment were found to exist between such criterion groups as nationwide samples of psychologists, psychiatrists and occupational therapists. Baker & Schulberg's study did not include data on the

Table 7-1
CMHI Scale Data for Criteria Groups*

Criterion Group	*N*	*Mean Score*	*S.D.*	*Range*
1. Harvard Postdoctorals	57	239.79	19.48	165-262
2. Harvard Visiting Faculty	15	234.60	26.91	160-264
3. Community Psychologists	23	234.43	14.68	195-264
4. Graduate Psychiatric Nursing Students	386	232.97	18.54	150-266
5. Social Work Students	105	231.75	20.12	154-257
6. Columbia Postdoctorals	25	221.96	24.06	173-260
7. American Psychological Association (Div. 12)	79	217.89	22.19	159-258
8. American Occupational Therapy Association	35	207.69	21.07	161-243
9. Soc. of Biological Psychiatry	29	206.28	32.97	131-258
10. American Psychiatric Association	175	198.93	37.02	92-265
11. American Psychoanalytic Association	46	194.52	31.23	125-259

*Data on criteria groups 1–3 and 6–11 are from Baker, F. and Schulberg, H.C. The development of a community mental health ideology scale. *Community Mental Health Journal*, 1967, *3*, 216–225; for criterion group 4 from Howard, Lucy A. and Baker, F. Ideology and role function of the nurse in community mental health. *Nursing Research*, 1971, *20*, 450–454; and for criterion group 5 from Penn, N., Baker, F. and Schulberg, H.C. Community mental health ideology and personality preferences. Unpublished paper 1973.

two major mental health professional groups of nurses and social workers, so that subsequent studies by the authors and their colleagues have been focused upon these disciplines. Howard & Baker (1971) obtained data from over three quarters of the graduate psychiatric nursing programs in the United States, with 386 psychiatric nursing students from 38 training programs completing CMHI Scales. Penn, Baker & Schulberg (1973) reported the results of administering the CMHI Scale to 105 social work students in four schools of social work in the Greater Boston area. The basic CMHI Scale data for the criterion groups on which the scale was developed plus the data on graduate psychiatric nursing students and social work students are presented in Table 7-1.

It is apparent in examining Table 7-1 that the ordering of the five professional groups is as follows: the two groups of students obtained the highest CMHI scores (i.e., graduate psychiatric nursing students and social work students) followed by the clinical psychologists, occupational therapists and psychiatrists. The two Harvard Community Mental Health criterion groups and the community psychologists who participated in the 1965 Swampscott Conference on Training in Community Psychology obtained even higher scores, but it is difficult to generalize to professional discipline from these exceptional criterion groups. Thus, our data suggest that psychiatrists appeared to be less committed to this new ideology than their nonmedical mental health professional colleagues.

The first study showing differences in orientation to community mental health ideologies among professionals working in the same organizational settings was reported by Langston (1970). Table 7-2 presents the merged means, standard deviations and ranges of CMHI scores for the major professional groups studied by Langston in his analysis of two Texas community mental health centers—one center established as part of a private general hospital and the other as part of a private psychiatric hospital. As in the Baker & Schulberg studies, Langston found psychiatrists to be the least committed to Community Mental Health Ideologies among the professional groups that he studied.

Table 7-2
CMHI Scale Scores of Texas CMHC Professional Groups Reported by Langston*

Group	*N*	*Mean Score*	*S.D.*	*Range*
Social Workers	9	235.89	16.41	200-257
Psychologists	7	229.00	20.36	185-248
Occupational and Recreational Therapists	20	213.65	16.82	180-255
Nurses	22	210.23	20.17	180-246
Psychiatrists	13	202.38	19.84	171-236

*Data presentation based on Tables 1 and 2 from Langston, R.D. Community mental health centers and community mental health ideology. *Community Mental Health Journal*, 1970, *6*, 387–392.

COMMUNITY MENTAL HEALTH IDEOLOGY IN A CHANGING STATE MENTAL HOSPITAL

As mental hospitals attempt to develop programs based upon a community mental health orientation, ideological controversies inevitably emerge among their staff members. Analysis of the patterns by which varying psychiatric ideological viewpoints are distributed among hospital staff, and of strength of ideological positions taken among and between work groups is vital for understanding the widely differing acceptance and development of community-oriented services within traditional mental health organizations. In an effort to learn more about the role of ideology in a traditional inpatient-focused mental hospital changing in the direction of more community-based activities, the authors undertook a study of the orientation toward community mental health ideology among Boston State Hospital staff.

Kotin & Sharaf (1967) described the ideology controversy existing in the hospital in 1965 following the arrival of a new superintendent who was perceived as more intent on developing social and community psychiatric approaches than had been his predecessor. The hospital's clinical staff was thought by Kotin & Sharaf to be divided between two ideologically distinct camps whose polarity was particularly manifested in the operation of the psychiatric residency training program. One group of clinicians favored a teaching emphasis upon psychoanalytic concepts and techniques which could produce individual personality change, even though this approach is applicable only to a selected number of mental hospital patients. Another group of clinicians endorsed the teaching of socially oriented rehabilitation techniques which are applicable to larger numbers of patients who can be treated quickly and discharged with minimal personality reconstruction.

A number of issues had been joined by 1967. In a variety of subjective ways the feeling had developed among observers that the hospital's staff had made a distinct ideological shift in the direction of community mental health concepts. The superintendent's differential reward policy of supporting staff who initiated innovative, community-oriented services in preference to traditionally oriented colleagues was beginning to have an impact. The hospital appeared to be moving toward greater ideological unity than had been true earlier, and it was deemed important to determine whether this was actually the case. Of particular interest was the question of relative adherence to community mental health concepts among different inpatient and outpatient work groups and among the various professional disciplines, since they are key elements affecting the hospital's ability to assume new caregiving functions. A study, therefore, was undertaken to objectively measure staff attitudes toward community mental health ideology. The results of this study, together with a brief case history describing the relationship of ideology to program development, are presented in the remainder of this chapter.

First Administration of CMHI Scale

The Community Mental Health Ideology Scale was distributed as part of a longer questionnaire to all professional staff who were working at Boston State Hospital in the month of May 1967, including physicians, psychologists, social workers, occupational therapists and registered nurses. Two weeks after the questionnaires were received by the staff, a followup letter was sent to nonrespondents, and after an additional two weeks had elapsed an attempt was made to contact the remaining nonrespondents either in person or by phone.

The overall response rate for professional personnel at Boston State Hospital was an acceptable 70.2 percent, as 177 of 252 such staff members returned completed questionnaires. The response rates of the specific disciplines (see Table 7-3) ranged from 56.1 percent among registered nurses to 100 percent in the BSH Psychology Department.

Table 7-3
Responses of BSH Professional Groups in 1967 to CMHI Scale

Group	*Number Administered*	*Number Returned*	*Percent Returned*
Physicians	91	67	73.6
Psychologists	15	15	100.0
Social Workers	37	30	81.8
Occupational Therapists	27	19	70.4
Registered Nurses	82	46	56.1

The CMHI Scale is keyed in such a manner that the maximum score of 266 indicates total and intense agreement with all facets of community mental health ideology (Baker & Schulberg, 1967). Analysis of the CMHI Scale responses by BSH staff indicates that in 1967 their total scores ranged from 142 to 264, with an overall hospital mean of 214.7, and a standard deviation of 28.0.

In addition to the overall hospital pattern, it is meaningful to consider the response distributions of each of the institution's five professional disciplines since they represent important power groups influencing policy change and program development. Table 7-4 indicates that as discrete groups, BSH social workers, registered nurses and psychologists had the highest mean scale scores and thus expressed the greatest adherence to community mental health ideology. The group means for hospital occupational therapists and physicians were considerably lower than those of the other disciplines although they were relatively high in terms of commitment to this ideology.

Are these differences among the five professional disciplines' CMHI Scale scores significant? Examination by means of a one-way analysis of variance (Table 7-5) indi-

Table 7-4
CMHI Scale Scores of BSH Professional Groups in 1967

Group	*N*	*Mean Score*	*S.D.*	*Range*
Social Workers	30	224.3	26.2	164-264
Registered Nurses	46	221.4	23.2	154-225
Psychologists	15	218.5	25.7	166-251
Occupational Therapists	19	208.6	23.9	142-249
Physicians	67	206.8	31.1	137-255

Table 7-5
Analysis of Variance of CMHI Scale Scores by Professional Group

Source	*MS*	*DF*	*F*
Between Groups	2489.85	4.0	3.36*
Within Groups	741.44	172.0	
Total	3231.29	176.0	

*$p < .05$

cates that in 1967 the five professional subgroups significantly differed in their ideological perspective.

The rank order of mean scores among the professional groups at BSH is somewhat different from that observed by Langston (1970) in his study of two Houston community mental health centers. The BSH professional nurses seemed relatively more committed to community mental health ideology when compared to their professional coworkers than the Houston nurses as compared to their coworkers. As was the case in Langston's study, the BSH medical personnel had the lowest CMHI Scale group mean. It is of interest to further divide the BSH physicians into a group composed of senior psychiatrists and a few senior psychiatrically oriented physicians, and to compare this group with psychiatric residents. The authors had found in their initial study with national samples that younger and more recently trained individuals tend to be greater supporters of community mental health ideology (Baker & Schulberg, 1967). Analysis of the BSH medical personnel subgroup scores indicated that the mean CMHI Scale score of 209.6 achieved by the 30 young psychiatric residents did not differ significantly from the mean of 204.5 achieved by the 37 senior psychiatrists.

The basic CMHI Scale statistics for BSH professional disciplines in 1967 (Table 7-4) were similar to those obtained by the random national samples of mental health professionals upon whom the scale was initially developed (Table 7-1). The mean total score of physicians at BSH (206.8) was not significantly different from the mean (198.9) of a random sample of American Psychiatric Association members. Similarly, the mean score of psychologists at BSH (218.5) was virtually the same as that obtained by a random sample of clinical psychologists in the American Psychological Association (217.9).

Second Administration of the CMHI Scale

Significant program changes and personnel shifts occurred at Boston State Hospital during the period subsequent to our initial administration of the CMHI Scale. The instrument was, therefore, readministered to hospital staff during April 1969 to determine whether the institution's ideological climate was changing, and if so, in what direction. The CMHI Scale was distributed to 263 psychiatrists, registered nurses, social workers, physicians and occupational therapists working at the hospital at the time. One hundred sixty-six completed questionnaires were returned in usable form, yielding a response rate of 63.1 percent. Table 7-6 shows that 67 of the staff members who had completed the 1967 questionnaire also completed it in 1969: i.e., 39.8 percent of the responses obtained in 1969 were from the same individuals who had completed the scale two years earlier. Table 7-6 shows the response rates and overlaps in the respondents from the five professional groups for the two administrations in the CMHI Scale.

The means, standard deviations and ranges for the second administration of the CMHI Scale to BSH staff (Table 7-7) indicate that the physicians, including psychiatrists, residents and other M.D.'s employed at the hospital, still had the lowest mean score on this measure of community mental health ideology. The rank order of means had changed since 1967; the mean

Table 7-6
Responses of BSH Professional Groups in 1969 to CMHI Scale

Group	*Number Administered*	*Number Returned*	*Percent Returned*	*Overlap With 1967*	*Percent Overlap*
Physicians	77	50	64.9	24	48.0
Psychologists	18	13	72.2	6	46.2
Social Workers	52	36	69.2	15	41.7
Occupational Therapists	30	24	80.0	7	29.2
Registered Nurses	86	43	50.0	14	32.6
Totals:	263	166	63.1	66	39.8

score for psychologists was now the highest while the mean score for social workers was now somewhat lower. Occupational therapists were still in fourth place but in 1969 had a mean ideology score closer to social workers than to physicians.

All groups, except for registered nurses and social workers, achieved somewhat higher average CMHI Scale scores in the second study. When the five groups are compared by an analysis of variance, it becomes clear that the differences which had existed among professional groups in 1967 have largely disappeared. An F Test shows statistical nonsignificance in the 1969 intergroup comparison (F = 1.61, p = .17).

The mean for all of the hospital's professionals on the CMHI Scale in 1969 was 216.69 as compared to the staff mean of 214.73 in 1967. Comparing scores for those individuals who completed this instrument both in 1967 and 1969, we found that the group means remained virtually unchanged over time (1969 mean = 213.47; 1967 mean = 213.25). However, in examining the scores of those individuals who completed the CMHI Scale only in 1967 but not in 1969, and vice versa, we found that the overall mean for the 1969-only respondents is significantly higher than that for the staff members who com-

Table 7-7
CMHI Scale Scores of BSH Professional Groups in 1969

Group	*N*	*Mean Score*	*S.D.*	*Range*
Psychologists	13	225.23	23.67	180-261
Registered Nurses	43	220.16	20.85	168-260
Social Workers	36	219.06	31.13	156-266
Occupational Therapists	24	218.33	30.12	115-255
Physicians	50	208.98	27.72	151-259

pleted the Scale only in 1967 (1969 mean = 219.3; 1967 mean = 205.1). The direction of the difference towards higher scores supports an interpretation that those professionals who joined the hospital's staff between 1967 and 1969 had stronger commitments to community mental health ideology than those who left the hospital during this time-period.

The data thus suggest that a selective rather than random leaving and entering of the system was occurring among staff. Individuals with a community mental health orientation were attracted to BSH and its new programs as an enticing work setting; those leaving the institution were more prone to view its new program directions as incompatible with their personal orientations. The subjective feeling of some observers that BSH was moving towards greater ideological cohesiveness during the late 1960s is supported by our finding that the significant difference in CMHI Scale scores among all professional groups which had existed in 1967 was not maintained in the comparison of 1969 scores across professional groups.

When the ideological orientation over time of specific BSH professional groups is considered, it is evident that psychiatrists and other medically trained staff continued to display the lowest average commitment to community mental health ideology among the five professional disciplines studied at the hospital. The psychiatrists' mean CMHI Scale scores in both 1967 and 1969 were comparable to that obtained by the national sample of members of the Society for Biological Psychiatry, one of the lower ranking criterion groups on which the Scale had been developed initially. Breeskin et al. (1972) had found a similar CMHI Scale mean score for the group of air force psychiatrists which they studied. An even lower score was obtained by Langston (1970) among the psychiatrists whom he studied in two Texas community mental health centers. Thus, the data which we obtained on the relatively low standing of BSH psychiatrists with regard to community mental health ideology commitment as compared to professional colleagues is not unique or exceptional.

On the basis of the relatively higher commitment found in several studies of nonmedical professionals to community mental health ideology, one would expect to find more support among these groups for program changes moving the hospital closer to its community. However, although nonmedical professions may dominate mental hospitals in terms of their sheer numbers, they do not dominate in terms of strategic placement within the hospital's decisionmaking hierarchy. This is perhaps one of the reasons why community mental health ideology finds relatively greater acceptance among nonmedical professionals; it emphasizes skills which are not directly dependent upon the usual training of medical professionals. Nonprofessionals in particular stand to gain in status if the ideas of the ideology are implemented. Even at BSH where some emphasis was given to the psychiatric treatment team approach and there was some implied promise of staff equality, it was clear that as is typically the case in organizations originally established upon the medical model, that medically trained personnel were more "equal" than other professionals.

THE INTERACTION OF IDEOLOGY WITH OTHER SOCIAL PSYCHOLOGICAL VARIABLES

The importance of considering the attitudes, values, beliefs and ideologies of the professional staff of a human services facility in conjunction with other sociopsychological variables and nonhuman resource variables in order to understand organizational behavior was stressed in Chapter 4. We noted that although attitudes and related human response disposition variables have been a central concern of social psychology since its inception, it has been difficult to show clear and direct relationships between the attitudes and behavior of individuals and groups. Only recently, however, have related investigations abandoned attitudinal variables as the sole basis for predicting behavior; attitude-behavior processes are now being studied as multivariate relationships. The view that attitudinal variables must be examined in the context of the numerous reality-based situational variables that shape behavior implies that individual response dispositions are simply one of the factors contributing to overt behavior decisions. Other relevant situational variables include the psychological, social and cultural influences in the action situation which combine to influence behavioral outcomes.

Acock & DeFleur (1972) describe the key to understanding behavior by means of attitudes as lying in "discovering interrelated configurations of attitude and social or cultural variables that accurately predict action [p. 715]." Behavioral predictions can be improved by combining attitude and social situational variables in a linear model based upon the interaction between these variables. Data were collected by Acock & DeFleur from 202 subjects regarding attitudes towards the legalization of marijuana, along with data on the subjects' perception of the position of peers and family. At a later date, subjects were observed in an experimental situation where they were asked to vote on the question of legalizing marijuana. Although a multiple regression solution showed that the independent effects of the three variables did not clearly predict behavior, their additive effect did somewhat better and the resulting configurations led to the clearest behavioral predictions. Thus.

Acock & DeFleur's results suggest that a configurational approach emphasizing the interaction of attitudinal and social situational variables can be an effective approach to examining the relationships of attitude and behavior.

The relevance of this multivariate conceptual perspective to the study of ideological influences upon mental hospital change was foreseen by Strauss et al. (1964). They identified three mechanisms that produce ideological differences among institutions, or between their subsystems: (1) variations in policy and procedure for the recruitment of professional personnel, (2) organizational variables such as resources, prevailing local patterns of treatment, and institutional necessity, and (3) opportunities and constraints for the feedback of practice into the formulation of refined ideological positions.

Strauss et al. also observed that persons with different ideological positions operating within similar institutional conditions emphasize different elements of the possible array of clinical services, and then organize treatment programs accordingly. Thus, although specific organizational and situational variables certainly influence the translation of ideology into treatment practice, other things being equal, ideology will make a difference in how professionals organize their working situations and approaches to treatment.

The relationship of community mental health ideology to program development is illustrated in the next section by a brief case description of the manner in which the differing community mental health orientations of two successive psychiatric directors of an outpatient clinic at Boston State Hospital affected the type of treatment services each sought to develop within the same institutional setting. Of particular relevance in this example was the clinic director's policy regarding such key community mental health concepts as a population focus, treatment goals and continuity of care. The director's role is emphasized because in situations of "medical dominance" (Freidson, 1970), the psychiatric director's ideology represents the predominant vector even though staff beliefs exert constraining influences.

Ideology and Program Development

The BSH Outpatient Clinic (OPC) was founded in the early 1950s and Dr. Adams,* who had taken a psychoanalytically oriented residency at BSH, became its director in 1959. He continued in this position until 1967 when he was succeeded by Dr. Green, a senior psychiatrist who had joined the clinic's staff the previous year. In contrast to Dr. Adams, whose CMHI Scale score of 205 was just about at the mean for BSH physicians, Dr. Green obtained a score of 233 which is almost a full standard deviation higher. In line with our hypothesis that ideology influences program direction, we predicted that the new director would introduce and support innovative community mental health-oriented services different from those of his more conservatively oriented predecessor. Data gathered over a period of two years after the change in directors appear to support our hypothesis.

Until 1964 the OPC was located off the grounds of BSH awaiting the construction of its new building. The primary function of the clinic was thought by Dr. Adams to be that of meeting the psychiatric resident's need to treat neurotics since experience on the inpatient services provided adequate opportunity to work with psychotics. "It is only in the outpatient program that the resident can learn to do longterm therapy with neurotics," contended Dr. Adams. Since only nonhospitalized

*Names have been changed.

neurotic patients were thought to be good candidates for intensive longterm therapy, alcoholics, drug addicts, court cases, psychotics and aftercare patients were all specifically excluded from the OPC as a matter of policy. The standing caseload ranged from about 120 to 150, and strict diagnostic limitations were enforced.

Even when the OPC moved into its new quarters on the grounds of the hospital in 1964, its service restrictions remained relatively unchanged. The clinic staff continued to perceive the OPC as an encapsulated subsystem within which high quality, intensive longterm therapy could by taught the residents through the admission of a small, selected number of patients. There was ongoing concern that the clinic's highly specialized work not be engulfed within the potential morass of the larger mental hospital. Indeed, even after BSH decentralized most of its patient services into semiautonomous comprehensive units in the fall of 1966, the OPC remained administratively and functionally separated from the remainder of the hospital's activities.

Dr. Adams resigned as director of the OPC in January, 1967 to spend all of his time in the BSH training program and he was succeeded by Dr. Green. Shortly after becoming the new director, Dr. Green indicated that he intended to make fundamental changes in the OPC's goals and services so that it would be better able to meet the needs of the community and be more fully integrated within other BSH programs. In accord with this orientation, Dr. Green quickly eliminated the OPC's restricted admission policy and advocated a policy of accepting for evaluation and treatment any individual living within the hospital's catchment area. Despite the constraint of having to develop new program directions with a resistant, veteran staff whose CMHI scale scores were even lower than that of Dr. Adams, it was possible for Dr. Green to implement major innovations in the OPC's work patterns. New patient assessment techniques began to be utilized, nonprofessionals were deployed among the traditional teams, a wider variety of treatment services was provided to patients and the clinic's total activities became integrated with the hospital's other subsystems. In fact, the function of evaluating any individual seeking inpatient or outpatient care at BSH was added to the clinic staff's responsibilities.

The question had been posed as to whether the assessment of one's ideological orientation alone is sufficient to explain major program modifications, or must we consider also the individual's position in his organization's hierarchical structure, the influence of environmental pressures for new services, and so on. Obviously, the changes which we have observed in the BSH outpatient clinic resulted from the complex interaction of all these variables plus many others but, nevertheless, an understanding of the director's psychiatric ideology was invaluable in more precisely defining his personal contribution to program development.

SUMMARY

Community mental health ideology has developed as a major belief system influencing program development in most psychiatric facilities. The impact of this ideology upon the staff of a mental hospital has been examined in terms of the patterns of commitment to community mental health concepts among different professional disciplines and work groups. Greatest support for this belief system was found among nonmedical professionals and the least among the nonprofessional members of the Nursing Department. A brief case example described the relationship of ideological orientation to program development in the hospital's outpatient clinic.

8. *Professional Roles and Relations*

The professional roles and relations of mental health workers have received considerable attention during the past two decades because we recognize that the effective operation of a psychiatric program requires the participation and cooperation of a number of disciplines. Various interaction patterns have evolved to meet this need for diverse skills, ranging from the simple availability, but separate functioning, of each autonomous professional group to relatively complex arrangements in which there is considerable sharing of clinical functions among all disciplines. Classic studies of these interaction patterns and the issues engendered by them were reported by Stanton & Schwartz (1954), and Zander, Cohen, & Stotland (1957). They found that although the mental health professions commonly value close teamwork, they also are organized in a definitely hierarchical manner. Psychiatrists, because of certain legal requirements and traditional practices, have the superior position and supervise the activities of other professionals, who often perceive themselves as subordinated.

Attention to the difficulties in developing and coordinating professional roles and relationships has intensified since the advent of the community mental health era. There is a pervasive concern with the appropriateness of certain functions for any given group and the nature of power as it is exercised or shared among the mental health team (Rushing, 1964; Grunebaum, 1970). This development is related to the previous failure to resolve many outstanding problems but is even more closely connected to the novel interpersonal complexities created for professionals participating in community-oriented caregiving programs based upon shifting ideologies.

Contemporary models of good professional practice require mental health workers to scrutinize their functions and skills with an intensity which potentially affects the fundamental roles they assume with each other. Equally significant demands are being made upon professionals to reassess the roles they assume and the relationships they cultivate with other caregivers in the community. The expanded roles of nonprofessionals and indigenous workers have further impacted upon changing interprofessional relations (Kaplan et al., 1970; Jacobson et al., 1970). In this chapter we therefore first will review the factors and trends affecting professional roles and relations in community mental health programs, and then analyze how these forces manifested themselves during a mental hospital's efforts to assume more community-oriented functions.

Role Ambiguity within the Mental Health Professions

A professional role can be defined as a specific set of behaviors concerning tasks which are expected of an individual by relevant others. These expectations define not only what the person must do but also how he must relate to others. Therefore, such dimensions as the power to influence decisions, relative knowledge and skills, and frequency of professional contacts are related to the individual's role in the organization. Some have assumed that because of the significance of professional roles, staff members of mental health organizations would carry out their functions with greater efficiency if each member were clearly aware of the characteristics of his own and others' roles. However, studies have shown repeatedly that considerable ignorance or ambiguity existed even before community mental health programs became prominent (Mill, 1960; Huber, 1963). Under these conditions of ambiguity, job satisfaction can be low, status rivalry high, decisionmaking poor, and patient care impaired.

To what degree is role ambiguity associated with the varying theoretical and practice models guiding community mental health programs? Programs based upon an organic and somatic etiological frame of reference generally have delineated clearcut roles for each discipline, with relatively little ambiguity as to the powers and responsibilities of each. The increasing adherence of community mental health programs to a socioenvironmental theoretical framework, however, has produced increased overlap of functions and role-blurring on the assumption that staff potential is maximized when disciplinary barriers are minimized. Although this is laudable in many respects, we must distinguish between constructive role-blurring which stems from an increased awareness of other disciplines' potentials, and destructive role-blurring based upon a desire to appropriate higher-value tasks or to pass on lower-value tasks. For example, a nurse might feel pleased when a psychiatrist offers her the opportunity to develop psychotherapeutic relationships with patients since this is a prestigious, high-value task. She might feel resentful, however, if asked to assume responsibility for violent patients since this could be perceived as "buck-passing" by the psychiatrist of a low-value task. Huber (1963) has described the confusion created by role-blurring in a therapeutic milieu and the fact that when one discipline expanded its role, another discipline's customary role was shared or even restricted.

A further complication of role-blurring in community mental health programs is the disparity created between a person's informal functions and the formal status assigned to his discipline in the interprofessional hierarchy. Personnel such as ward attendants may be told by nursing administrators that their clinical services are equal in importance to those of all other team members. Yet they receive lower salaries, have less opportunity for advancement, and see daily multiple evidences of their lower status.

Sensitive interpersonal issues arise at the present time from the interracial composition of many urban mental health center staffs, and incidents of prejudice are intertwined with interprofessional status differentials. Alleged discrimination related to sex also has become a prominent issue in mental health centers utilizing personnel in flexible, nonroutinized ways. Problems of differential status are particularly acute in those programs organized on the flexible and untraditional human services model described in Chapter 2, and it is doubtful that psychiatrists will indefinitely retain leadership of them on the basis of title rather than on relevant administrative skills and patterns of functioning. Similarly, it will be difficult to justify and maintain the discrepancy in pay scales for the different disciplines if community mental health programs continue to espouse role-blurring and the sharing of responsibility.

We also must recognize that interprofessional relations are affected not only by the the role definitions established within the organizational work group—that is, the clinical team—but also by the standards and values of local and national professional groups. It is not unusual for these different frames of reference to conflict, and the individual is faced with the necessity of selecting the model which best meets his immediate or longrange needs. For example, the member of a newly decentralized clinical service is often torn between an earlier allegiance to the department head who is a member of his own discipline, and the present relationship with his clinical team leader who comes from a different discipline. The more novel the interprofessional model developed within the work group, the greater the likelihood that it will conflict with the more conservative, established standards of the several professions. Familiar examples can be cited of the discomfort experienced by mental health professionals when required to assume new roles and divest themselves of traditional ones because of uncertainty as to whether they are being disloyal to their colleagues and professions (Bonn & Kraft, 1963; Baker, O'Brien, & Sheldon, 1968). Thus, the flexibility and creativity desired within new community programs are unfortunately constrained by conservative national norms; but, fortunately, national norms inevitably are modified by the novel interprofessional experiences emerging from various centers around the country.

TRENDS IN INTERPROFESSIONAL RELATIONS

As new models of community-oriented mental health service delivery continue to develop, several trends have significantly affected the evolving patterns of interprofessional relations. These trends include: (1) changes in the structure and composition of mental health teams; (2) changes in generalist-specialist functions of mental health staff members; (3) changes in leadership based on individual competence rather than membership in a particular professional discipline; and (4) changes in interprofessional relations stemming from systemic arrangements in which agencies work together on a coordinative, equalitarian basis rather than in a hierarchical pattern of organization. Each trend will be discussed separately although each is obviously interdependent with the others.

Structure and Composition of Mental Health Teams

The term "team" when used in mental health organizations is replete with ambiguity. Jepson (1970) notes that "the term team means different things in different settings; it is not simply the usual trinity of psychiatrist, psychologist and social worker [p. 461]." As a working unit, the interdisciplinary team is seen by some as crucial to the community mental health center's goals of providing a comprehensive range of services and continuity of care. Levenson (1970) states emphatically that, "in order to have an effective center program, it is necessary that the staff members function as a team and that team work extend to all aspects of the center's program [p. 552]."

The concept of the clinical professional team existed in mental hospitals and other psychiatric institutions long before the advent of community mental health centers, and while "team" implies cooperative endeavor, such work units historically have not always acted in harmony to produce better patient care. In analyzing the application of the "team concept" in psychiatric agencies, Hirschowitz (1973) has observed that this work pattern is sustained by a series of myths. One myth is that "in team decision-making, democratic process obtains." Hirschowitz, who himself is a psychiatrist, candidly observes that in reality every team in a psychiatric setting actually has a hierarchy of power and influence. The physician-psychiatrist, because of his ascribed status and his "medical responsibility," expects and is expected to assume a disproportionate share of responsibility for both the team's decisions and their outcome; the physician thus maintains a dominant hierarchical position. Hirschowitz emphasizes that nonphysician team members covertly accept and reinforce the existing dominance hierarchy in order to avoid the risk and responsibilities of shared or delegated decision-making.

The subtleties incorporated within the dominance hierarchy in the psychiatric team veil another assumption which Hirschowitz describes as mythical, i.e., "the psychiatric team, because it pursues truths, permits untrue statements to be challenged." Hirschowitz asserts that decision-making within a psychiatric team is actually skewed; only individuals occupying a superior position in the organizational hierarchy are free to challenge the clinical opinions of lesser-ranking participants. Team members in a "one-down position" because of their disciplinary affiliation and lower hierarchical status are not free to question the conclusions or assumptions of a person in a superior position without running the risk of sanctions for insubordination. Since the nonphysician members of the psychiatric team typically occupy a lower position in the hierarchy, prevailing "truth" relates primarily to the opinions of the physician-psychiatrist members of the team.

The clinical professional team, thus, is either a major potential source of disharmony and inefficiency in community mental health programs, or a meaningful work unit upon which to build contemporary services. Disunity or disagreement within the team can have a negative effect on the patient, while in those situations where a team works effectively and achieves open and frank communication there is the distinct possibility of improved patient welfare.

In a case history of changes in the work climate of a residential treatment center for children, Kempler (1971) describes the development of effective teamwork and the achievement of improved interdisciplinary cooperation over the course of three years by means of "communication meetings" between the treatment staff and administration. The team moved towards greater group cohesion and better working relationships among individuals with different professional statuses, philosophies and experience. Kempler describes the positive changes as resulting both from regular meetings which encouraged the open expression of feelings, as well as the congruence of the changes with staff values and needs. The leadership of the ward administrator and the milieu coordinator provided an important initiating impetus and sustained support for the achieved changes.

The composition of mental health teams is being modified as programs become more sensitive to social concerns and the effects of poverty, racism and urban life. Certain professionals are consequently experiencing shifts in their levels of influence and prestige, particularly in human services programs. Despite intense conflicts between professionals and "nonprofessionals" of the type described by Shaw & Eagle (1971), some of the groups now in a marginal status with respect to their degree of professionalism, such as neighborhood case aides, have taken advantage of opportunities to further advance their identity by establishing more formal criteria of accreditation, thus securing a stable place for themselves in the mental health field (Vidaver, 1973). The modification of mental health teams through the addition of settlement house workers, probation officers and other such agents is another, probably painful, transition which will particularly affect human services–oriented programs. The dismay expressed some years ago by a psychiatrist such as Jacobson (1967) about the "boldness of some inadequately trained persons in attempting to see patients . . . with the sanction of clinic directors" continues to reflect the inner sentiments of many other mental health professionals, and continued conflict can be expected because of blurred roles and overlapping domains of activity. Less difficulty is encountered in medical-practice programs because of their clear stipulation of the psychiatrist's prerogatives and responsibilities.

Generalist-Specialist Functions

The growth of community mental health programs has increased the need to clarify the nature and extent of the generalist and specialist functions of each mental health team member. Even though these two functions are in many ways antithetical, the aim of well-developed training programs has been to present workers with a core curriculum that allows them to be maximally integrated with other professional groups while at the same time retaining their own professional identity and skills. In terms of actual practice, mental health workers usually maintain their specialist skills, such as administering psychological tests or prescribing medication, within their own center, but they function as generalists in dealing with a community's total range of needs via consultation activities. The difficulties which such a dichotomy engenders are not always easily resolved. Rosenblum & Ottenstein (1965) reported that at one of the first community mental health centers to adopt this work pattern, staff members who engaged in extensive community consultation soon were viewed as lobbyists overly identified with the narrow interests of a particular geographic area. To maintain the balance needed in a comprehensive program, it became necessary to impose a limit upon the amount of time that any staff member could spend in generalist community activities if he was still to fulfill his specialist clinical responsibilities.

Leadership Based on Individual Competence

The development of community-oriented mental health programs has nourished the viewpoint that program leadership should be based upon individual competence rather than upon membership in a particular discipline. For many years administrative responsibility has been assigned primarily on the basis of arbitrary criteria such as degree and discipline, with resultant disharmony and ill-will toward the traditional leader, the psychiatrist. Many social workers and psychologists have often turned to social agencies and universities as settings in which they can aspire to leadership without being confined by the narrowly circumscribed hierarchy of the mental health agency.

To some extent, this trend has been reversed and valuable manpower is being retained in community mental health settings by growing attention to Yolles's early reminder that nowhere in the federal regulations about community mental health centers was it suggested that administrative leadership be limited to psychiatrists (Yolles, 1966). In fact, the changes made in the regulations on June 7, 1967, stated, "The overall direction of a center may be carried out by a properly qualified member of any one of the mental health professions." Although the principle of individual competence rather than professional prerogative has remained a point of contention in many local medical practice model programs, it is being implemented in those programs emerging from a social and community-oriented practice model. By 1973, the American Psychiatric Association had adopted the principle of administrative leadership based upon individual competency as its policy for community mental health programs, and this progressive national policy inevitably will affect local standards and practices.

Interagency Relations

Personnel in caregiving facilities commonly perceive interagency relationships in terms of hierarchical patterns of organization. Some agencies are viewed as more prestigious and dominant, others as less significant and influential. An operational equilibrium develops, however, over time and, correctly or incorrectly, psychiatric directors of new community mental health programs often are viewed as threats to the systemic status quo. Local anxieties are particularly heightened by fanciful statements that every aspect of community life has significance for mental health and, therefore, is subject to the psychiatrist's review.

The medical practice model has tended to reinforce interagency suspicions more than the human services model since the former implies that psychiatrists have the responsibility and perhaps even the power to organize the community's total mental health program. Greater concern for interagency relations is reflected in the human services model, which emphasizes that effective operation of the community's program requires coordinated and equalitarian rather than hierarchical working patterns among participating personnel. Thus, careful attention must be given to cultivating positive relationships between agencies' staffs as well as among personnel within the mental health center itself; "role-trespassing," i.e., assuming another group's previously accepted unique functions, is destructive in either instance. The management of this complex dimension of interagency professional relationships can be even more difficult than resolving the familiar problem of intracenter staff relationships, and it behooves mental health professionals working in the community to be particularly aware of its subtleties and consequences.

Professional Roles and Relations at a Changing Mental Hospital

The reviews in Chapters 5 and 6 of Boston State Hospital's modified program directions and altered administrative structure, as well as the following two chapters on the hospital's environmental contacts and clinical services, clearly indicate that controversial issues about professional roles and relations both abetted and constrained these developments. For example, the preceding and succeeding analyses detail the anxieties and tensions generated among psychiatrists and psychiatric residents in the face of changing programmatic emphases which blurred their unique functions and traditionally superior status. In a similar vein, Duhl (1971) has presented a remarkably personalized and frank description of his aggressive efforts to align Boston State Hospital's psychiatric residency training program with the institution's evolving community mental health ideology. The resistances among both his psychiatric and nonpsychiatric colleagues stemmed from local as well as national ambiguities about program standards and work functions.

The role modifications and professional dilemmas encountered by Boston State Hospital's other disciplines as they groped for solutions to the turmoil of organizational change have received less attention in this volume and, again, in the general mental health literature. We, therefore, have chosen to focus our analysis of roles and relations in the community-oriented mental hospital upon the issues which confronted occupational therapists and psychiatric nurses during the selected periods of our study. Both disciplines had responsibilities vital to the organization's new program aims, and they were instrumental in stimulating and performing therapeutic patient-care activities. The occupational therapists' tasks were crucial to the rehabilitation of hundreds of chronic patients whom the hospital wished discharged. Psychiatric nurses were at the fulcrum of the hospital's several decentralization plans intended to improve acute patient care. How these two professional groups perceived Boston State Hospital's changing program directions and adapted their roles to them will be considered in the remainder of this chapter.

THE OCCUPATIONAL THERAPIST'S REFERENCE GROUPS

A professional's selection and perfecting of work tasks appropriate to his role usually are conducted in relation to his reference group orientation, i.e., the group or groups with which he identifies and looks for normative standards of behavior. It often has been demonstrated that professional workers in bureaucratic organizations are confronted with conflicting role definitions, and that they are prone to develop either a "local" or "cosmopolitan" orientational pattern. Those adopting the local pattern are more oriented to the standards of the organization in which they work and give major consideration to its expectations in defining personal tasks; those adopting a cosmopolitan orientation tend to give primacy to the expectations of external groups such as their profession and colleagues in other work settings.

The community-oriented program activities already evident at Boston State Hospital when our study began in 1965 led us to analyze the role orientations of occupational therapists to determine whether they were compatible or in conflict with new organizational directions. Five groups whose norms and expectations could affect the daily work tasks of the hospital's occupational therapists were identified. These were the total hospital organization, the work group (the group of fellow hospital staff with whom the occupational therapist works in treating patients), the profession of occupational therapy, the local geographic community and occupational therapist colleagues at the hospital.

The first two groups may be considered as internal reference points, and the second two as external reference points. The fifth group, the hospital's occupational therapy department, although existing within the organization's boundaries, may be considered as an intermediate frame of reference. It combines a mixture of intraorganizational and extraorganizational commitments, depending upon the degree to which it stresses professional concerns in contrast to emphasizing organizational production functions.

A questionnaire study was undertaken to determine which reference groups dominated and influenced the work orientation of the psychiatric occupational therapists at Boston State Hospital. We were also concerned with how these orientation patterns related to the previous work experiences and education of such staff persons. Questionnaires were distributed to the hospital's entire complement of 26 therapists at an occupational therapy department meeting in the spring of 1966. We explained that code numbers were being employed to ensure confidentiality of individual responses, and staff were asked to fill out and return questionnaires to us in sealed envelopes collected at the occupational therapy department office. Nineteen of the 26 occupational therapists returned their questionnaires within a period of two weeks.

The questionnaire contained randomly distributed, forced choice statements comparing the significance of each of the five reference groups with every other one in relation to patient-oriented work tasks. The resulting 10 pairs of comparisons were arranged so that each reference group appeared first in the statement as often as it appeared second. Staff responses were made on a six-point agree-disagree scale indicating slight, somewhat and strong agreement or disagreement. Accompanying the "Occupational Therapist Reference Group Scale" was a cover sheet asking for personal information regarding age, time at hospital, work experience in occupational therapy and education.

The staff's responses for each statement contained in the questionnaire are presented in Table 8-1. By examining the total number of "agree" and "disagree" responses to each question, a quick indication is obtained of the respondents' feelings toward each of the five reference groups. It is immediately clear that the hospital work group is a meaningful reference point and affects the occupational therapist's work tasks; her fellow group of Boston State Hospital occupational therapists is a relatively unimportant frame of reference for determining patient-care tasks. However, this global comparison does not consider the respondent's *relative* commitment to each reference group vis-à-vis her commitment to other groups. We, therefore, utilized an overall index score which took into account the respondent's choice of one reference group over another as well as consider-

Table 8-1

Occupational Therapists' Reference Group Choices in Working with Patients

Reference Group Pairings	*Responses:* *Agree*	*Disagree*
(1) In working with patients, the standards of the profession of occupational therapy come before the needs of this hospital.	7	12
(2) In working with patients, the needs of Boston State Hospital as a whole must be considered before the needs of one's work group.	8	11
(3) In treating patients, the needs of the work group must come before the standards of the profession of occupational therapy.	10	9
(4) In treating patients, the needs of the group of occupational therapists at Boston State Hospital are more important than the standards of occupational therapy as a profession.	8	11
(5) In working with patients, the standards of the profession must be considered before the needs of the community at large.	8	11
(6) When working with patients, the needs of the hospital as a whole are more important than the needs of the group of occupational therapists at Boston State Hospital.	13	6
(7) When working with patients, it is more important to consider what is needed by the work group than what is needed by the community at large.	14	5
(8) In treating patients, the needs of the community at large must come before the needs of the group of occupational therapists at Boston State Hospital.	12	5
(9) When working with patients, the needs of the group of occupational therapists at Boston State Hospital must take precedence over the needs of one's work group.	2	17
(10) In treating patients, the needs of the community at large must be considered before the needs of Boston State Hospital.	5	14

Table 8-2
Occupational Therapists' Choices of Dominant Reference Group
(N=19)

	Internal Groups		Intermediate Group	External Groups	
	Work Group	*Hospital Group*	*OT Group*	*Professional Group*	*Community Group*
Choices	9(47%)	2(11%)	0(0%)	4(21%)	4(21%)

ing the strength of response.* The index score was totaled for each possible reference group, and the group receiving the highest score was considered to be the individual's dominant frame of reference.

The distributions of reference group choices based upon the index score indicated that for approximately half of the occupational therapists, the internal work group was primary in patient care decisions. The two external reference groups, i.e. the profession of occupational therapy and the local community, were the next most frequently chosen reference points, followed by the internal hospital group. No occupational therapist chose the intermediate reference group of fellow Boston State Hospital occupational therapists as dominating her orientation to the treatment of patients. The distribution of scores among the five reference groups is presented in Table 8-2.

*The index score for each group was computed for every respondent by the formula developed by Berkowitz (personal communication).

$$I = \frac{X_1(X_1 \cdot LX)}{\Sigma X} \Sigma D$$

I = Index score, X_1 = Absolute value of group in question, LX = Lowest value of five groups, D = Discrepancy between values.

In calculating the index, strong agreement or disagreement was assigned a value of 3; "somewhat agree" or "somewhat disagree," a value of 2; slight agreement or disagreement, a value of 1.

The relationships between patterns of internal and external orientation and professional experience were investigated by comparing the dominant reference group choices of staff members whose work experience in occupational therapy was greater than one year, with those whose experience in occupational therapy was one year or less (one year being the median length of work experience for the 19 respondents). Table 8-3 presents the distribution of internal and external reference group choices for respondents at these two levels of experience. Respondents with longer work experience in the profession of occupational therapy chose internal reference groups significantly more often than did those with shorter work experience.

The length of time an occupational therapist had worked at Boston State Hospital was also related to her choice of dominant reference group. Staff who had worked at the hospital for more than the median time of one year chose the internal reference groups significantly more often than did staff who had worked at Boston State Hospital less than one year.

Neither a person's total education, including occupational therapy training, nor her age were found to be

Table 8-3
Length of Time as Occupational Therapist
and Reference Group Orientation
(Internal vs. External)

Time as Practicing Occupational Therapist	*Reference Groups Chosen*	
	Internal	*External*
More than one year	8	1
One year or less	3	7

Significant at p = .025 by Fisher Exact Probability Test

Table 8-4
Time of Occupational Therapy Training
and Reference Group Orientation (N=9)

Time of Training	*Reference Group Chosen*	
	Internal	*External*
Pre 1957 Training	5	0
Post 1957 Training	0	4

Significant at p = .01 by Fisher Exact Probability Test

significant factors in choosing reference groups. However, the time at which a person completed her training in occupational therapy was a significant element in selecting reference groups. Considering the 1957 academic year following the Allenbury Conference on Occupational Therapy Education as the dividing point, we found that persons trained since that time were oriented toward external reference groups while those trained prior to that date were oriented toward internal reference groups (see Table 8-4).

Our data indicating that the work group was the dominant reference point for the largest number of Boston State Hospital occupational therapists is consistent with the earliest studies of worker motivation and control. For example, Bennis et al. (1958) found that the work group is a prime dispenser of rewards and punishments for a nurse's actions in the treatment of patients. Similarly, the occupational therapist spends the majority of her working hours in the company of a functional work group, and it is understandable that multidisciplinary colleagues exert a powerful influence upon her patient treatment orientation. While other occupational therapists at the hospital comprise a peer group of the same occupational rank, they are not adjacent to her in the work-flow structure nor is there any evidence of direct contact among occupational therapists during their work with patients except in the relatively rare situation where two occupational therapists are members of the same work group. Therefore, the role-setting capabilities of fellow hospital occupational therapists are not as potent as those of the work group.

The underchoosing of fellow occupational therapists at Boston State Hospital as a dominant reference group in determining patient care tasks does not indicate that the occupational therapy department is without influence. On the contrary, the department's efforts were directed toward helping the occupational therapist define her role as both a member of the treatment team—i.e., the work group—and as a member of the profession of occupational therapy. In our interviews with the two heads of the department, the goals of the service were outlined by its leaders as those of increased involvement in community mental health programs and strengthened professional identity among the staff. Thus, our findings are consistent with the department's policy of not arbitrarily restricting an occupational therapist's functions, but rather reinforcing the view of the occupational therapist as an integrated member of the psychiatric treatment team.

The questions had been posed of how the work experiences and education of occupational therapists affect her choice of internal or external reference groups. The most clearcut finding was that therapists trained since the time of the national Allenbury Conference were in all cases primarily oriented toward the external reference groups of the profession and the community; those educated earlier looked to the internal reference points of work group and hospital group for principal guidance in defining role behavior in the treatment of patients. For an administration pursuing new program directions, what are the implications of (a) this finding, and (b) our data that respondents with more experience in the profession of occupational therapy and with more experience at Boston State Hospital are more internally oriented in selecting patient care tasks?

We infer that it is the differential socializing effects of recent education versus experience in a traditional mental hospital which accounts for the different reference group orientations evident among our respondents. Occupational therapists educated since the Allenbury Conference have been socialized to act as members of interdisciplinary treatment teams in programs whose functions may well extend beyond the boundaries of the hospital. For example, at the time of our study at Boston State Hospital an occupational therapist was creating a pioneering role for her profession on the hospital's home treatment service (Weiner et al., 1967). Her work tasks included assessments of patients' functional capacities and the prescribing of remedial programs relevant to the patients' home settings. On the other hand, occupational therapists principally socialized to professional roles within traditional mental hospitals are more comfortable within hierarchically structured, multidisciplinary work groups, and they limit their patient-care tasks to hospital-based shops and clinics.

Thus, it seems clear from our data that a hospital administration attempting to reorient the institution's goals and functions away from traditionally internally focused concerns towards a community mental health perspective would gain greater support from more recently educated, less experienced occupational therapists than from earlier educated, more experienced personnel. The former are more committed to external reference groups with compatible contemporary orientations; the latter are more influenced by internal reference groups whose activities are the very target of change.

In summary, this case example has examined two sources of influence on the occupational therapist's role orientation—the influence of internal and external reference groups, and the impact of training and experience. These factors were suggested to be key determinants of the occupational therapist's ability to assume new work tasks consistent with the hospital's movement towards community mental health concerns. Furthermore, the fact that the occupational therapy department sought to exert but a minor influence upon its staff's choice of specific patient care tasks eased the ability of these professionals to function comfortably within the new decentralized unit structure described in Chapter 6. The unique functions of each unit's work group therefore became an even more dominant influence upon the occupational therapist's professional role while her discipline's central department assumed staff rather than line functions in the unitized mental hospital.

A Centralized Nursing Department in a Decentralized Hospital

Boston State Hospital's increased orientation to community mental health goals and its adoption in 1966 of the decentralized unit system had a far more disturbing and profound effect upon the nursing department than upon the occupational therapy department. In contrast to the latter group, which readily accepted the hospital's internal unit work groups as the prime reference points for defining job roles, nursing administrators maintained their cosmopolitan orientation towards the nurse's role. They deemed external professional norms to be as crucial as organizational ones for determining a nurse's tasks.

The nursing department also was loath to relinquish administrative and supervisory control over its personnel, despite the hospital's movement toward a decentralized management structure. For some time, the department continued to function as a powerful professional subsystem with traditional line responsibilities rather than new staff ones and, thus, generated much controversy among the other disciplinary and clinical subsystems, which had adjusted to the hospital's decentralized structure. Baker et al. (1970) have reviewed the administrative problems created when one subsystem maintains centralized functions within a decentralized organization. We now will consider efforts of the nursing department's leadership to maintain professional roles geared as much to external reference groups as to internal ones and the implications of such efforts for multidisciplinary work groups.

The Unitization of Nursing Staff

We had noted in Chapter 6 that a key requirement for the mental hospital's decentralization is adequate personnel to staff each newly established unit. This necessity is particularly acute as it regards nursing personnel since only the professional and nonprofessional members of this group are physically present and responsible for a unit's operations 24 hours per day, seven days per week. The dilemma of how optimally to distribute Boston State Hospital's limited nursing staff had been a key concern of the organization's leadership as it pondered adoption of the unit system. Directors of three of the four proposed units sought increased nursing staff while the director of the fourth proposed unit insisted on retaining his relatively large complement of nurses.

When the superintendent decided in August 1966 to unitize the hospital, a plan developed by the director of nursing for distribution of his personnel among the units was agreed upon. The plan was based upon a continued centralized nursing department retaining authority to reassign staff vacancies among the units and to approve the requests of nurses who voluntarily sought transfers. A more equitable pattern was established accordingly and no nurses were forced to relocate against their wishes.

Pursuing the traditional model of medical authority, a senior psychiatrist was appointed as head of each of the four units and given the responsibility for developing a clinical program along whatever directions he considered appropriate. Few restrictions were placed on the autonomy of the newly developing units. In fact, common unit problems around patient care acted to bring members of different occupational groups in closer contact with each other and less with fellow members of the discipline. As a consequence, a unit's multidisciplinary staff often banded together in competition with other units for scarce organizational resources. Identification with and loyalty to the unit were also reinforced by the administration's frequent references to unit-based psychiatric treatment teams. The concept of a "team," with its implied egalitarianism, naturally was very appealing to nonpsychiatrists in a hospital which for years had operated under a medically dominated administrative structure.

As the geographically oriented units gained program strength and identity, the role of professional departments was increasingly challenged. The training of psychiatric residents remained under a clear, centralized authority; however, the centralized departments of nursing, social service, psychology and occupational therapy assumed increasingly ambiguous positions in the hospital's organizational structure. The nursing department's retention of centralized authority over its personnel's deployment and functions became particularly controversial since the shortage of nursing staff continued unabated. It seemed to even intensify as units cared for both acute and chronic patients. Unit chiefs began to question the nursing department's practices with regard both to the allocation of vacant positions and to the recruitment, hiring, and deployment of nursing staff. Frequent demands were made to turn these functions over to the unit chief on the assumption that individual unit programs would thus fare better.

The Nurse's Planned Role

Under pressure from a number of sides, the centralized nursing department continued to examine its role and functions in the decentralized hospital. About six months after the initial unitization, the director of nursing developed a plan for the "functional reorganization of the nursing department" into three divisions: administrative, clinical and education. Each division was to be headed by an assistant director of nursing, who together with the director, comprised the nursing executive board.

The complex plan established three different lines of nursing authority for each unit. Under the overall supervision of the assistant director for administration, each decentralized service was assigned its own senior administrative supervisor who held line authority over the unit's R.N.'s, ward charges, L.P.N.'s, and attendant nurses. The assistant director for the nursing department's clinical division supervised senior clinical R.N.s and clinical specialist R.N.'s on each unit. Finally, the educational division was comprised of an assistant director-coordinator R.N. and senior instructor R.N.'s who were assigned to individual units.

The development of a caseload for clinical R.N.'s was viewed by the nursing department as a central purpose of its new plan, and this staff function was elaborated as follows:

> Their nursing practice responsibility is to divide the existing inpatient population in their units into caseloads, pick up new patients on admission on a rotating basis, write up nursing care plans in conjunction with the medical care plan for their caseloads, collaborate with administrative personnel in carrying out the nursing care plan, provide individual and group nursing therapy to patients, as appropriate, coordinate other hospital and community resources toward the restoration of the patient to his maximum potential.

The nursing department asserted that nursing caseloads were a creative clinical innovation intended to foster the professional growth of nurses as well as to provide the best possible nursing care for all patients. The caseload systems developed at other mental hospitals were pointed to as models, and consultants were invited from a small rural private mental hospital to discuss the development of their particular program. Licensed practical nurses and attendant nurses were not considered to be a part of such a clinical division. Clinical functions for "nonprofessional" nurses were specifically excluded from the plan.

The nursing department's administrative division was assigned the task of maintaining a therapeutic milieu for patients, carrying out the physician's medical care plan and collaborating with the patient's clinical nurse in implementing a nursing care plan. Thus, members of the administrative division were seen primarily as aiding both the doctors and clinical nurses and as maintaining the ward environment. Clinical work on a one-to-one basis was excluded from the job tasks of this division's nurses.

The responsibilities of the educational division were to "develop an appropriate inservice program for all levels of nursing personnel, collaborate with administrative and clinical supervisors in the assignment of students for clinical practice, share with the administrative and clinical supervisors in establishing nursing policies and practice in the respective units, plan for workshops and conferences and coordinate nursing educational services."

The nursing department's plan made the R.N. responsible for specific patients whom she would follow through all stages of hospitalization and aftercare. The L.P.N. would cease to perform clinical tasks and increasingly would take the role of a ward administrator, thus freeing the R.N. from ward admission duties so that she might spend more time with patients. In general, the plan was thought to offer the following advantages for the nursing department and the entire hospital:

1. It would provide better clinical care since each patient would have a specific nurse assigned to him. There would be greater continuity of professional services, including aftercare where possible.
2. It would clarify the nurse's role.
3. The reorganization of the nursing department would aid the nurse's professional role development.
4. It would allow the development of individual nursing staff potential.
5. It would increase the hospital's reputation as an innovative facility and thus attract new nursing staff.
6. The reorganization of the nursing department would complement the hospital's unitization and would "allow nursing to assume greater responsibility as a

member of a therapeutic team involved in the newer trends of community psychiatry."

Putting Plans into Practice

From its very inception, the nursing department's plan generated considerable controversy and encountered opposition among both nursing and non-nursing personnel. The department's director was the target of much personal criticism. Others perceived him as unwilling to cooperate with the hospital's decentralized structure and as wishing to maintain a nursing "empire." The lingering tensions produced by unitization among all personnel as they adapted to unit work groups was focused upon the nursing staff which maintained strong linkages to its central department. Consequently, the multiple stresses associated with the nursing plan's implementation outweighed its projected advantages, and it ultimately was dropped. In retrospect, the following factors seemed to militate against successful adoption of the nursing director's design for new nursing roles in a decentralized hospital:

1. Identification with the reorganization plan and its goals. Few nurses at Boston State Hospital saw the caseload system and the clinical-administrative split of nursing roles as goals with which they could personally identify. Most continued to view the reorganization of the nursing department as basically the "director of nursing's plan." Those who felt positively toward the director tried to implement the plan in order to please him; a few of the newer staff who shared his goals for expanding the professional role of nurses worked very hard at trying to make the plan work. Those who personally felt negatively toward the director of nursing expressed their resentment through passive resistance to his scheme.

2. *Departmental cohesiveness.* A related impediment to the plan's adoption was the lack of cohesiveness within the nursing department, a situation which had existed even before unitization. The hospital's large size and the differentiation of its services among widely separated buildings, as well as the lack of a regular and continuing forum for bringing together nurses from different clinical units worked against a strong identification with the nursing department. We noted earlier that our study of the reference group orientations of the hospital's occupational therapists found that OT staff, particularly those who had been at the hospital more than a few years, tended to identify more with their work groups than with their professional department. A similar situation seemed equally true among nurses, and this pattern was evident in data collected through a "reference group orientation scale" administered to a small sample of nurses.

3. *The splitting of nurses' roles.* A fundamental feature of the nursing plan was its effort to assign distinct and nonoverlapping tasks to departmental personnel. However, nursing supervisors expressed much discomfort about the "administrative-clinical split," contending that it was arbitrary and unnatural. This issue continued as a topic of heated discussion at the department's newly formed policy and practices committee throughout the year following the plan's introduction. Although the "split" had been presented to nurses and accepted by some of them as more clearly defining nursing tasks, in practice the change only seemed to further confuse the nursing staff's roles. For most of the staff unitization had not created any major change in physical surroundings or in the technologies of patient treatment, but it had produced altered relationships with other members of the work group. Since many nurses had not been

able to clarify the personal implications of modified interprofessional relationships, the simultaneous reorganization of nursing department functions had only intensified ambiguity and confusion about nursing roles.

A basic premise for the splitting of nursing tasks was the recognition that "some people are more talented than others in some areas and could better be used this way." The reorganization plan offered the department's leaders an opportunity to assign nurses to roles where they could better employ unique experiences, skills, and interests. Additionally, by highlighting the clinical division of the nursing department and its concern with clinical work tasks, the department thought it could attract young college-trained persons who had been educated to perceive the nurse's role as a clinical professional. On the other hand, the role of administrative supervisor would allow older diploma-school nurses, who had been at Boston State Hospital for many years and who had come up through the ranks, to attain positions of status in which they might utilize their greater knowledge of ward management procedures. But the reality, as one supervisor summarized it, was that:

> At this hospital we cannot afford the luxury of only one talent. The clinical supervisor was supposed to be more concerned with clinical problems and patients but she often held herself apart from the ward.... Often the nursing supervisors are not really qualified.... Through longevity a head nurse sometimes makes supervisor. She is taken out of a situation where she is doing well and put into another place because there is no other system of rewards.

Implementation of the split nursing role also was hindered by the fact that the plan's paper distinctions among the tasks assigned to the clinical, administrative.

and educational supervisors were obscured in the unit's daily operations. Nurses met great difficulty in assigning practical responsibility and authority among the three supervisors. In some units the role of educational supervisor and clinical supervisor tended to overlap. Both L.P.N.'s and doctors were confused about which supervisor they should deal with in regard to specific ward problems. Furthermore, only one supervisor might be present when the problem arose and conflicting decisions were sometimes made. The situation was described by a nurse in this way:

> When the administrative supervisor is on, she will make one certain policy. When the clinical supervisor is on and a problem comes up, she would make a different policy, since she is not aware of the first policy. When the administrative supervisor returned, she wonders why the policy is different.

Finally, the intended benefits of the plan's split assignments turned out to be counterproductive because old antagonisms were intensified by the confusion and competition for status. Most nurses felt that the role of clinical supervisor offered more prestige, and some administrative supervisors expressed resentment at giving up their clinical patient-care responsibilities. The latter group was particularly upset by the appointment of younger, recently graduated nurses as clinical supervisors. Those nurses who gained in status as the result of the new appointments naturally viewed the promotion with favor, but even they were uncomfortable about their new role's lack of clarity.

4. Inadequate numbers of professional nursing staff. The nursing plan's division of responsibilities among the professional and nonprofessional members of the department was intended to attract newly trained personnel with strong clinical interests. However, the hospital's chronic problem of unfilled professional nursing job blocks continued unabated after the plan was undertaken, and few new applicants were immediately recruited by the splitting of nursing functions. In fact, the formal transfer of "nonprofessional" nurses from clinical responsibilities to ward management tasks further limited the staff available for direct patient-care services. The L.P.N.'s and aides in the clinical division felt alienated from the nursing department, since they no longer were considered "professionals," and some turned to the labor union that was developing in the hospital as a new reference group which would support their interests. An administrative supervisor noted that the plan "shook the nonprofessional staff. It increased their responsibility and decreased their authority." Another supervisor added, "The L.P.N.'s don't want to be called 'ward administrators'; they want to be called L.P.N.'s. They want to be treated as nurses, which they are."

5. *Resistance of medical staff.* The decentralization of Boston State Hospital had placed greater importance upon the unit work group and its activities as a frame of reference defining each discipline's role and tasks. The aspirations and professional interests of any one discipline increasingly could be satisfied only in relation to the desires and work habits of colleagues from other disciplines. Thus, the nursing department's wish to implement a plan establishing clinical specialists among its staff depended not only upon the acceptance of this format among administrative nursing personnel, but also upon the cooperation of psychiatrists since medical care plans were to be used as basic models of nursing care. The clinical nurses were instructed to "write up nursing care plans in conjunction with medical care plans and

provide nursing therapy appropriate to the needs of the patient." Too often, however, the nurses found no psychiatric patient care plans on which to base nursing plans.

In seeking such medical guidelines and publicly emphasizing their absence, clinical nurses may have created further antagonism among unit psychiatrists towards their new roles and responsibilities. Implementation clearly was hindered as psychiatrists tended to ignore the new lines of authority created by the nursing department for its personnel. Rather than respecting the new nursing assignments, psychiatrists preferred to work either with the ward nurses they liked personally or whoever happened to be available at the time. In one unit, the chief psychiatrist was so perturbed with the new young graduate nurse appointed clinical supervisor that he didn't even speak to her; instead, he issued his directives through nurses on the evening shift.

6. Nurses' unwillingness to fight physicians. It has been observed that professionalism requires a more militant stance than most women traditionally have been willing to assert in hierarchically structured organizations. The nursing director at Boston State Hospital found that the majority of the female nurses were reluctant to actively work for the implementation of his plan in the face of medical opposition. Although most of the nurses did not openly oppose the nursing director, by the same token, neither did they actively support him in his dispute with the medical staff which regarded the nursing plan as antagonistic to customary interprofessional relations and task assignments. The director of nursing thus found himself torn between the conflicting need to support his nurses at the decentralized work group level as units gained power, while at the same time trying to retain his own central control in order to pursue what he perceived to be the needs of the total hospital. Not surprisingly, he soon felt that he was not being supported by his staff, and chided nurses for their reluctance to speak up in disputes with doctors. After a year of attempting to hold the nursing department together in the face of its staff's growing identification with work group units, the director of nursing expressed his dismay and frustration as follows:

> There doesn't seem to be an identity of purpose. There doesn't seem to be any transcending of units. We've become too unitized. There's a lack of identity, considerable miscommunication, and discord within and between units. This doesn't lead to good feelings in the nursing department. There is strong feeling against having a nursing department. Maybe we should just have units.

The nursing plan's complexity, novelty and controversial nature ultimately produced its demise. Disheartened by opposition among nurses and non-nurses, the nursing department director resigned his hospital position in 1968, and the department soon turned to more decentrally oriented procedures for integrating nursing roles with those of the other disciplines.

Generalist and Specialist Roles

As mental hospitals move from traditionally inpatient-focused services towards a broader community orientation, what is the effect upon the customary tasks of each mental health discipline? Our review of how Boston State Hospital established geographically based, decentralized units indicates that multidisciplinary work groups tend to blur narrow, specialist roles and stimulate generalist functions. For example, some psychiatrists and nurses began to move hesitantly into increased contacts with the community, occasionally causing social workers to express concern about "unwarranted" encroachment on their traditional area of specialization. Similarly, the psychiatric director of the hospital's outpatient clinic assigned responsibility for interviewing and evaluating those seeking service to young "clinical specialists," who often were college graduates with personal aptitude but little experience. Naturally, psychiatric residents felt devalued by what they perceived as role trespassing upon a significant medical function.

The reactions of a mental health discipline to the generalist trend will vary in relation to many national and local concerns. Overt responses must be understood as stemming also from historic as well as immediate circumstances. When such an analytic framework is utilized, the rationale for and efforts of Boston State Hospital's nursing director to counter his organization's generalist trend become clearer. Long subjected to a subordinate role designed primarily in keeping with physicians' needs, the nursing department's staff seized upon unitization as an opportunity to create specialist tasks of their own. Intent to establish internal performance standards and to control personnel deployment, the nursing department ironically turned to psychiatry's familiar but not totally applicable model of the practitioner-client relationship and adopted it as its own.

The nursing director, who was quite active in national nursing associations, attempted to justify this plan to the hospital staff by avowing that in order to provide better patient care it was important to move toward a more professional—i.e., specialized—role for nurses and "to bring to Boston State Hospital what goes on in the nation with regard to nursing." Most of the hospital's psychiatrists, and nurses as well, did not view this assertion as adequate justification. They feared that the nursing plan would detrimentally affect the multidisciplinary, generalist team system that had been started with decentralization, a goal of greater significance than specialized nursing roles. There seems little doubt, then, that although nursing staffs nationally (Howard & Baker, 1971) as well as that at Boston State Hospital (Geyerhahn & Mesnick, 1971) have moved towards a community mental health orientation and embraced a generalist view of the nurse's role within such programs, the director of nursing at this institution remained committed to an earlier professional framework which stressed the specialized role development of nurses as psychotherapists with inpatients.

SUMMARY

The functioning of any system is dependent upon the role differentiation and integration which management develops among those responsible for meeting the organization's production goals. In this chapter we have described some of the problems of changing professional roles and relationships within a mental hospital evolving in the direction of greater community-oriented tasks. While the multidisciplinary team may be seen as crucial to the community mental health center's goals of providing a comprehensive range of services and continuity of care, this functional concept is not without inherent ambiguities and difficulties. Case examples of changing occupational therapist and nursing tasks have been presented as illustrations of the problems related to generalist and specialist definitions of professional roles, and the potential conflict provided by competitive orientations to either internal or external reference groups. There can be little doubt but that the tasks traditionally deemed inviolate by each discipline will continue to be altered, and that the specialist functions of previous years will be viewed as generalist ones in the future.

9. *The Mental Hospital and Its Environments*

Much thought and action have been directed in recent years to the key task of how best to relate mental health programs to their communities. Recognizing the need for mental health services which assume a more interactive, less isolated stance vis-à-vis their environments, citizens and professionals have devised various interorganizational patterns for better linking psychiatric facilities and their communities. As a result, the mental hospital has experienced particularly dramatic changes in its types and degree of extraorganizational contacts as it has moved from a condition of rural enclave into the urban milieu. The traditional arrangement whereby the large psychiatric institution was isolated, and isolated itself, from its surrounding community has been replaced by a system of linkages which permit the mental hospital to assume contemporary functions. In the process, the mental hospital has been forced to relinquish some of its autonomy, but, more significantly, the larger community has developed a stake in the activities and fate of the hospital and its patients.

An earlier review by Greenblatt & Schulberg (1970) described the many community linkages relevant to the mental hospital's primary goals of good patient care, the training of new professionals and the conducting of research. These linkages are becoming increasingly diverse as they involve the public, voluntary and private spheres of community life. Newly cultivated relationships with private foundations have generated fresh funds for demonstration services, and other recent linkages have similarly expanded the organization's ability to convert difficult inputs into satisfactory outputs, e.g., utilizing foster families to house chronically ill individuals in the community. From a systems perspective, it should be noted that the growth of certain interorganizational relationships can adversely or positively affect the development of others. The increased reliance of voluntary mental health agencies on governmental bodies for fiscal support has sometimes constrained the agencies' flexibility in negotiating linkages with other components of the nonpublic sector because of contractual restrictions. Conversely, many of the new interaction patterns are complementary and reinforce each other's development. The increased contacts between mental health programs and educational systems have permitted the former to obtain significantly growing support from manpower development sources, and the latter to play an emerging role in the creation of new professional careers.

With these considerations about the complex character of community linkage patterns in mind, this chapter will first review the general nature of organizational environments and then consider the specific community systems relevant to the mental hospital's goals of patient care, professional training and psychiatric research. We will then focus upon the mental hospital's links to preventively oriented community-based activities since they keenly illustrate the issues affecting the institution's capacity to function as a community mental health center.

ORGANIZATIONAL ENVIRONMENTS

Organizations as living systems differ from nonliving systems in their greater openness to and interaction with the external environment. We noted in Chapter 4 that the planners and managers of program change must, therefore, consider not only the internal variables affecting progress but also those environmental vicissitudes capable of hindering or abetting transitional efforts. Panzetta (1971) has suggested that a community has at least four levels of confrontation that it can mobilize: (1) as physical force, (2) as antiparticipant, (3) as franchiser and (4) as consumer. Providers of community mental health services must perceive their proper relation to these forms of confrontation. The process is further complicated by the fact that environmental contexts are becoming increasingly complex, and themselves subject to change as the result of organizational transformations.

The variety of differing environmental conditions within which mental hospitals and most human services organizations function have been classified by Emery & Trist (1965) into four ideal types, and arrayed on a continuum according to degree of certainty-uncertainty and interdependence exhibited among the component parts or sectors. According to this schema, society may be viewed as moving from the one extreme, in which conditions affecting program development were relatively placid and randomly distributed, to the opposite extreme, in which ever more complex interconnections and fluctuating forces confront organizations with "turbulent" environments. The turbulence has been created by expanding scientific and technological developments, by changing societal values, by altered professional domains and, perhaps most notably, by people's growing aspiration to control rather than to be victims of their surroundings. The mental hospital's environment has been drastically altered and enlivened by psychopharmacological successes, by society's increased tolerance for mental illness, by the growing use of nonprofessional personnel and by expanded citizen roles in determining program priorities.

Each of Emery & Trist's four ideal types of environment differs in terms of the behavioral predictability it offers to the mental hospital relative to the structures and forces in its environment; each type, therefore, requires a different organizational strategy for coping with external developments. Adaptation is easiest in the placid environment and can proceed by trial and error without threatening organizational viability. Mental hospitals stumbled for many decades through appropriate and inappropriate program efforts and, nevertheless, survived. During turbulent periods, however, survival and continued organizational autonomy are dependent upon an ability to generate sophisticated plans and strategies for obtaining goal consensus and relevant resources. The mental hospital of the 1970's must be capable of assuming a future-oriented stance, anticipating changed societal standards of psychiatric care, and negotiating its role and level of fiscal support within a complex framework of competing human services caregivers. An inability to master these tasks could lead to the hospital's demise. It is evident, then, that as environments change, organizations must alter interaction patterns with their surroundings so as to produce a better "fit" with external demands. The mental hospital in the era of community mental health has been required to design new and specific boundary-spanning subsystems capable of dealing with community concerns. We now will consider the variety of linkages relevant to the mental hospital's assuming contemporary functions within a turbulent environment.

Governmental Regulations and Support Systems

Most American mental hospitals are publicly financed and operated as units of some larger governmental structure which ultimately derives its authority from legislative mandates. Regardless of whether the hospital's links to the legislature are of a direct or indirect nature, the organization must always be mindful of legal statutes since they affect its assigned scope of activity, geographic catchment area, personnel utilization patterns, etc.

The legislature impacts upon the mental hospital by establishing public policy, as seen, for example, in its regulation of admissions procedures to this facility. For many years, the institution's patient inputs consisted primarily of individuals legally committed to its care, thus reflecting the environment's desire for a relatively closed hospital system with carefully regulated inputs as well as outputs. Changed social values and the community's increased ability to accept the mentally ill within its midst have led legislatures to approve voluntary admissions procedures. The mental hospital's functions, inputs and outputs have changed accordingly. Entrée to this psychiatric facility no longer need be a quasilegal matter for most of those seeking its care, and discharges have been similarly simplified and eased.

It is clear, however, that although the legislative and professional systems currently agree about the merits of a voluntary admissions policy, future differences may arise between the two systems since they adhere to somewhat differing social values. In fact, some professionals feel that they must vigilantly guard against legislative tendencies to proscribe professional standards and practices. Nevertheless, our current ethos is such that most professionals accept the public's right to assert a monitoring function, and standard-setting mechanisms of varied restrictiveness are being established. An ongoing dialogue between the legal and professional viewpoints must, therefore, be maintained, a process crucial to the mental hospital's ability to experiment with pioneering procedures and fresh roles in patient care.

The need to obtain and maintain adequate financial

support is a further area in which the mental hospital is linked to the community as represented by the legislature. As one of many competitors for the limited tax dollar, the hospital with close relationships to the legislature is likely to fare best in generating vital monetary inputs. The sophisticated administrator, therefore, will expend considerable effort in developing positive rapport with his community's legislators. The maintenance of this link is furthered by the recognition of all participants that just as the hospital administration must appeal to the legislature for support, so do legislators require favors from the hospital for their constituents. Judicious use of this quid pro quo linking strategy has often enhanced a hospital's ability to highlight its unique needs and pioneering services to maximum fiscal advantage.

The community mental health era has placed even further significance upon hospital-legislature working relationships since many new federal grant programs have required a matching component from local funds. Federal community mental health staffing funds are granted only if the organization demonstrates the ability to assume total support for personnel after a period of several years. The public mental hospital, thus, must negotiate a tripartite agreement between itself, the federal agency and the state legislature before it can benefit from such additional financial inputs.

EDUCATIONAL AND PROFESSIONAL SYSTEMS

Most modern mental hospitals view the training of new mental health professionals as one of their major goals and, therefore, strive to establish community linkages which will permit achievement of this objective. Inputs from the community, i.e., trainees and teachers, long have been sought from the universities and medical schools. Such linkages have permitted the hospital to keep apace of advancing knowledge, but additionally the affiliations have afforded the hospital staff the prestige and recognition associated with the university environment. The tighter the linkage that the hospital has cultivated with the university, the more secure has become its academic, training and research climate.

In the past the mental hospital usually was forced to take the initiative in seeking out universities which would be interested in exploring mutually beneficial relationships. Increasingly, however, universities themselves have come to recognize the advantages of affiliating with mental hospitals. Through such a linkage the university can gain rich diversified clinical material for its teaching needs, greater flexibility in operating biological and social laboratories and, frequently, physical space for expanding research enterprises. With the present uncertainty created by federal cutbacks in training program support, universities have come to view mental hospitals additionally as providing support for training faculty and students. Greenblatt (1965) advocated joint appointments of qualified staff to both the hospital and university, joint commitments to salaries, and joint training and research programs as the accepted standards of an alliance between the mental hospital and the university. Although unfeasible in certain instances, these standards have become routinely accepted in many other liaisons between the clinical and educational systems. Fiscal pressures may well insure that they are applied to training linkages as well.

Although linkages have long existed for the training of mental health professionals, we now are witnessing a rapid diversification of the hospital's relationships with academia. Not only do ties exist for the training of psychiatrists, psychologists, social workers, nurses, etc., but also for such professions as lawyers, city planners, political scientists, theologians and public relations counselors as well. Beyond the university system, the mental hospital is also developing links with its local elementary school network. Through this relationship the hospital can obtain the special education teachers so vitally needed for its total rehabilitative effort directed at emotionally disturbed and retarded youngsters. As the scope of the mental hospital's interests has broadened and people's awareness of the varied forces affecting the mentally ill has grown, ever-expanding linkages have been generated between the psychiatric facility and the community's educational institutions.

Very much related to the mental hospital's evolving links with the educational system are the ties which it must maintain with national and local professional societies. A growing source of concern for the mental hospital as it attempts to secure these links is the fact that each of these professional groups is struggling with new role-definitions and seeking higher status in our rapidly changing world. Furthermore, as the mental hospital diversifies its technological system for treating patients, nonpsychiatric professional groups acquire greater leverage in their competition for a place in the mental health sun and thus reinforce the interprofessional struggles in which they already are engaged (Schulberg & Baker, 1970; Vidaver, 1973). As the functions and structure of the mental hospital continue to be redefined, previously reluctant professional societies have approved legislation permitting the appointment of lay mental hospital administrators so long as medical responsibility for patient care remains vested in a psychiatrist. Community mental health legislation at the federal and state levels of government is authorizing the appointment of many types of mental health professionals to such key positions as directors of community mental health centers, regional directors, assistant commissioners and even commissioners. Since the treatment of mental patients continues to involve diverse specialty groups, the mental hospital obviously must continue to maintain appropriate links with the professional system of each group represented on its staff.

In this regard, we are often prone to overlook the crucial role played by the community's labor organizations in determining mental hospital personnel policies. These labor groups, which particularly represent the many members of nursing departments and nonclinical work groups, may be branches of the state AFL-CIO or they may be local associations. It is through them that individual grievances are presented, and it is with them that general policies for working conditions are administered. Labor's approval and cooperation are imperative for inaugurating new programs which necessitate altered demands on personnel, and in modifying civil service regulations so as to permit such far-reaching administrative powers as transferring staff from hospital wards to community-based settings.

Research and Development Systems

The mental hospital will encounter overwhelming competition for trainees of all disciplines unless it can offer them a vigorous research environment within which to pursue studies along a broad range of interests. To build such a milieu the hospital must be capable of attracting the familiar triad of men, money and materials, and the techniques for doing so have been of central concern to many administrators. Indeed, institutions have even recruited "grantsmanship" specialists to help in the quest for financial inputs so that research operations can be expanded.

Few linkages existed in the past between the mental hospital and community outlets for research funding. Research was largely confined to university laboratories or associated medical-surgical teaching hospitals since financing was primarily through university funds. However, the geometric growth during the 1960s in the federal financing of research greatly broadened the types of institutions eligible for such funds, and it has produced profound changes for the mental hospital interested in research.

More recently there has been a dramatic proliferation of agencies and resources that in some form contribute to mental health-related research. Sources outside the National Institute of Mental Health, formerly the mental hospital's prime supplier of research and development funds, have dwarfed that institute in their significance for the hospital. As the problems of poverty, social deprivation, delinquency, addiction, alcoholism, aging, corrections, etc., emerged in their centrality to our national welfare, the mental hospital has been advantageously positioned to receive relevant new funds because of its lengthy experience with and time-honored service to the poor and indigent. As national thinking increasingly embraces the relevance of man's total ecological context for his happiness and well-being, the mental hospital with diverse research interests will have varied opportunities to pursue and establish appropriate funding linkages in the community.

Mental hospitals which increasingly emphasize research and development experience profound changes in the climate and operation of their organization. Not only must space and budgetary allowances be made for these activities, but considerable time must be expended in the recruitment of personnel, cultivation of foundations, brainstorming of new ideas, preparing applications for support and reporting past progress. Thus, many mental hospitals formerly dominated by the routines of clinical activity have now become vital laboratories for human investigation with a creative and intellectual climate rivaling that of academic centers.

CITIZEN SYSTEMS

Environmental systems of a governmental, educational or developmental nature possess relatively clearcut relevance to the mental health professional, so that linkages between these systems and the mental hospital have readily developed along many of the previously described pathways. The purposes of linking psychiatric institutions to the community's citizen systems remain more ambiguous and controversial, however, and patterns of meaningful citizen-institutional ties continue to evolve in ambiguous if not contradictory ways.

The mixed nature of these contemporary links is ironic and in marked contrast to bygone eras, dating back to the nineteenth century, when citizen bodies constituted an established formal channel through which the public's viewpoint could be injected into the hospital's operation. Such groups as boards of trustees or visiting committees were statutorily authorized to exercise significant degrees of control over program direction, and they wielded considerable influence as spokesmen for their communities' social values and service priorities The rise of professionalism and increasingly technologically oriented treatment modalities diminished citizen linkages and inputs during the twentieth century, and by the 1950s, the public's ties with psychiatric institutions were more perfunctory than real.

The need for direct citizen involvement in setting program goals and priorities is a key concept of community mental health ideology. With the growing adherence to this orientation beginning in the mid-1960s, vigorous and protracted debates have ensued between lay boards and mental health professionals as to the primary locus of power and program control. The various state community mental health acts passed in recent years range in philosophy from those giving citizen boards complete budgetary and administrative control to those in which the citizens' links to program design and operation are primarily advisory in nature.

Mental hospitals maintaining an intraorganizational focus place a low priority upon initiating or accepting overtures from community citizen systems. However, institutions seeking to expand clinical, training and research activities into the local environment have been challenged as part of this effort to modify insular professional controls, and to establish more open working relationships with citizen systems. The complexities and vagaries of determining optimal "community involvement" are key negotiating issues as professionals and their lay counterparts seek consensus about this concept's definition, its rationale and operational parameters. Bolman (1972) has identified several inevitable difficulties in the quest for professional-lay rapprochement: community participation, once begun, can move rapidly toward community control; programs may change in ways that professionals will question; issues of racism and sociopolitical ideology intensify disputes and make them more complex; and legitimate differences over goals create unavoidable irrelevant conflicts which impede constructive change. A failure to resolve these problems can lead to the type of volatile upheaval experienced in 1969 by the Lincoln Hospital community mental health service. Among the reasons cited by Shaw & Eagle (1971) for Lincoln Hospital's "programmed failure" was its failure to abide by a commitment to community control. They assert that "when values were really tested by the exigencies of money and power, the colonial and racist attitudes prevented . . .the professional management of the program from being able to see the community as being capable of taking responsibility for its own affairs [p. 263]." The problem of how best to involve citizens remains critical but unresolved, so that further experimentation with optimal linkage patterns most likely will continue in both fruitful as well as controversial directions as the mental hospital seeks to refine this vital tie to its community.

CAREGIVING SYSTEMS

Although it is possible to define relatively clearly the manner in which each of the essential services in a community mental health program should be provided, the organization of these elements into a comprehensive system is a far more formidable problem. In many communities it isn't feasible, or even wise, for a single facility to provide the full spectrum of required services by itself. Certain elements of the comprehensive program may already be provided through agencies other than the mental health facility, and duplication would be not only wasteful but also deleterious to interagency cooperation. It therefore is necessary and much more practical for a combination of existing and possibly new agencies to coordinate their programs in such a way that the community obtains a complete range of services.

In practice, the human services caregiving system in most communities is usually a loosely organized set of agencies, institutions and professionals that individually pursue their own goals and interests but collectively look after the sick, indigent and disturbed. In the case of the mentally ill, coordinating linkages have developed between the mental hospital and numerous community caregivers in such manner that patient inputs to and outputs from the hospital are significantly related to the nature of these linkages. Indeed, the pattern of these ties can be viewed as a prime determiner of the types of people who enter and leave the mental hospital. The following are some of the key linkages in the community's formal and informal caregiving system with which the mental hospital must constantly negotiate a viable relationship:

1. *Those individuals recognized by the community as appropriate channels of appeal in the case of mental disturbance.* Included in this group are not only medical practitioners but also clergymen, lawyers and police. A significant proportion of inpatient and outpatient admissions to the hospital have long been funneled through these individuals, and an increasing number are being returned to the community with their assistance. General practitioners, in particular, have become increasingly involved in the medical management of discharged patients.

2. *Social welfare agencies.* A broad variety of agencies exist for the treatment and management of problems which are centrally or peripherally related to mental illness. These community agencies include family service centers, child guidance clinics, settlement houses, multiservice centers, rehabilitation offices, etc. The mental hospital's services for its patients are vitally affected by the referral and treatment policies of these agencies since they are in a position to determine the volume and types of patients sent into the hospital as well as to assist in aftercare arrangements for those individuals whom the hospital wishes to discharge. These organizational relationships have been particularly stimulated by the

federal community mental health regulations (HEW, 1964), which require contractual arrangements among appropriate caregivers so as to insure continuity of patient care.

3. *Other medical and psychiatric hospitals.* The local general hospital, the veterans' hospital, and the private psychiatric hospital provide a significant volume of service to a community's mentally ill and thus inevitably interact with the mental hospital. The expansion of psychiatric units in general hospitals has been a particularly crucial development during the past decade. In those communities where such facilities exist, admission patterns to mental hospitals have been significantly modified. Acute depressive and schizophrenic reactions frequently are treated in the general hospital while geriatric and organic problems still are referred to the mental hospital. A related medical facility of significance for the hospital's capacity to output patients is the nursing home. In recent years it has become a major albeit controversial resource in the care of chronic patients; as an alternative inpatient facility it has been instrumental in reducing the mental hospital's census.

4. *The legal and correctional network.* A growing part of the mental hospital's services are directed towards its community's legal and correctional programs. A significant number of patient admissions are conveyed to hospitals by the police, while the courts regularly request psychiatric opinions regarding the sanity and antisocial behavior of its clientele. To meet this need for collaborative effort with the criminal justice system, mental health facilities have developed an elaborate network of linkages which is perhaps most clearly centered in the burgeoning specialty of forensic psychiatry. Seminars in forensic psychiatry are being offered by the mental hospital

to various correctional and legal personnel as part of the hospital's effort to generate and sustain interaction patterns with this key segment of community caregivers. Such activities are particularly necessary in the light of evolving court decisions which emphasize the treatment of the criminally insane in mental hospitals rather than penal institutions.

5. *The family and family surrogate system.* Perhaps the most vital of all the links which the mental hospital must forge in the community is that with patients' families. After many decades of benign neglect, institutions have turned to families with the realization that the relatives' involvement is a key factor in determining length of patient hospitalization and adjustment after discharge. Indeed, much of the chronicity so evident in mental hospitals today is the result of having permitted families to detach themselves physically and psychologically from the relative who required intensive but temporary inpatient care. Family involvement is being achieved through a variety of administrative and therapeutic approaches. Some psychiatric programs will not even admit the patient unless the family agrees to participate in the treatment process. In other instances, the patient's family is encouraged to participate in conjoint diagnostic and therapeutic interviews through a home service treatment-type of arrangement before admission. The participation of families is particularly vital for those patients treated in a day hospital if they are to remain at home evenings and weekends.

In those instances where the patient's family is unavailable, uncooperative or even antitherapeutic, the hospital has devised surrogate family groups to serve as the vital interpersonal, community-based link. Realizing the necessity for providing individuals with satisfactory experiences in family living, the hospital has long worked with foster families and more recently with halfway houses as community resources capable of filling this major need. The success or failure of family surrogates in reintegrating their patient members to community living appears to be very much related to the selection of proper "parents" who are stable, flexible, and nourishing, and the selection of patients who wish to use the experience constructively rather than destructively.

It is obvious from even this brief description of the community mental health caregiving system that in most communities a wide array of linkages are potentially available to the mental hospital wishing to expand its interaction patterns with other local agencies. The question arises, however, as to how the participants can best relate in an integrated network so that patient care is enhanced while interorganizational strife is minimized. This question has become an increasingly serious one with the simultaneous proliferation of agencies meeting diverse human needs and the shrinking fiscal base for supporting all of these efforts. It is clear that duplication of effort and coordinated services are luxuries which can no longer be afforded and that integrative mechanisms must be devised. Cumming (1971) has suggested that from a sociological point of view the following issues will have to be faced and resolved before the existing inefficient methods for delivering psychiatric services are improved: (1) the possibility of replacing the present stratified, categorical system of separate services for the rich and the poor with a single system; (2) central v. local control of auspices, funding, administration and program delivery; and (3) whether psychiatrists are medical specialists or gurus. It is unlikely that these issues will be uniformly resolved throughout the country, but rather that each community will achieve unique solutions based upon local precedents, the characteristics of role incumbents with potential boundary-spanning functions, the nature of the broader environment within which the total caregiving network operates and the specific type of psychiatric facility being utilized.

Despite the unique nature of each community's solution, it still is possible to detect common underlying features in the patterns selected for achieving program integration. In Chapter 2 the major contemporary systemic patterns were identified as: (1) the medical organizational network in which the mental health center views pathology as primarily an intrapsychic process and seeks to organize those community resources capable of providing necessary medical and/or psychological treatment; and (2) the human services network which views the etiology of mental illness as strongly rooted in pathological environmental conditions so that the mental health center cultivates linkages with all resources capable of ameliorating these adverse forces. The latter model has gained increased consideration during recent years, and Demone's (1974) analysis of these developments highlights the opportunities available to mental health centers participating as components of human services networks to insure comprehensive programs and continuity of care.

The model developed by a mental hospital for interacting with other community caregivers may change over time, and within large, complex organizations may even assume sharply differing characteristics at the same time. Thus, some decentralized units of a large psychiatric institution may arrange for extensive formal exchange of patients and resources with affiliated neighboring agencies, while other units of the institution may engage in little such activity. Some units may restrict their community relationships to those caregivers skilled in the psychiatric tasks of intensive care and rehabilitation, e.g., clinics, hospitals, and sheltered workshops, while other components of the same organization may cultivate interaction patterns specifically intended to further primary prevention goals, e.g., joint efforts with antipoverty agencies and model cities programs.

Finally, it is well to emphasize Baker and O'Brien's (1971) caveat that interorganizational coordination is sought because of an implicit assumption that such linkages are the intervening variables between human/material resource allocation and "effective" or "comprehensive" human services. This assumption has rarely been empirically tested. It is possible that "coordinated" human service organizations might in certain circumstances produce a less optimal mixture of outputs than those produced by organizations jealously seeking to further their own individual goals in competition with neighboring agencies.

BOSTON STATE HOSPITAL AND ITS ENVIRONMENTS

This chapter's analysis of the ways in which the environment and its various caregiving subsystems stimulate and constrain a mental hospital's program will now be applied to our study of Boston State Hospital's evolution into a community mental health center. The hospital's relationships with the catchment area's health and social welfare network will be reviewed, and we then will consider the factors abetting and hindering the hospital's efforts to develop a preventively oriented neighborhood service center closely linked to the surrounding community.

Many community mental health catchment areas seem gerrymandered because their boundaries are determined by arbitrary administrative criteria rather than sociological concepts of community. We had noted in

Chapter 5 that the area designated for Boston State Hospital by the 1966 Massachusetts Community Mental Health Act had little unity and was heterogeneous on all relevant variables; its geographic sections differed widely in racial and ethnic composition, resident mobility, socioeconomic status, etc. The Dorchester-Mattapan component was enmeshed by turbulent racial change and increasing poverty. On the other hand, the West Roxbury, Roslindale and Hyde Park segment consisted of stable, white middle-class neighborhoods whose population had increased almost 10 percent from 1950 to 1960 while the city of Boston's population was decreasing 13 percent during the same decade. Overt social pathology was less evident in "West-Ros-Park" than in tension-ridden Dorchester-Mattapan, and the former's contacts with Boston State Hospital had been minimal. In contrast to Dorchester-Mattapan, which sent the majority of its mentally ill to the public mental hospital, residents of West Roxbury, Roslindale and Hyde Park were heavy utilizers of private and V.A. hospitals (Massachusetts Mental Health Planning Project, 1965). Thus, the total catchment area assigned Boston State Hospital was a quite diverse one, requiring that the hospital design unique programs to meet the specific needs of its differing sections. The hospital's contacts with the catchment area's residents and caregiving organizations over the years had ranged from minimal to extensive but, clearly, new linkages had to be developed in the mid-1960s, even in the Dorchester-Mattapan section where the involvement had been heaviest.

Community-oriented mental hospitals, as a particular type of human services organization, function as open systems whose basic components are comprised of people along with beliefs and resources. Boston State Hospital for many decades had functioned as a medical institution concerned primarily with providing societally mandated inpatient services to highly troubled individuals. It is not surprising, then, that in the mid-1960s hospital-community interaction patterns determining patient input and output followed limited and narrow rather than multiple and flexible channels. Thus, during the first six months of 1965, more than half of the hospital's Dorchester inpatient admissions were individuals transferred from local general hospitals and citizens brought in by the police. Few admissions could be identified as emanating from the community's social welfare network. Furthermore, the majority of Boston State Hospital admissions during this time-period had been involved with court commitment proceedings; only 7 percent were of the voluntary type, despite the growing national acceptance of this medicolegal procedure.

Perceiving itself to have relatively little control over the organization's inputs—i.e., the types and volume of community residents seeking inpatient care—the hospital's staff exerted considerable energy in developing a more flexible network of resources for its outputs— i.e., treated patients to be returned home to the community. Local agencies had been fearful of accepting a discharged psychiatric patient for aftercare services, and many of the hospital's social workers and nurses went to considerable lengths to demonstrate the backup support which they would provide agency staff. There was, however, a considerable backlog of uncertain and negative experiences which had to be overcome before full cooperation would be obtained (Baker, Schulberg & O'Brien, 1969). Public welfare workers hesitated to accept referrals, since they felt untrained to cope with the behavior of psychiatric patients and feared that they would be left holding the bag, particularly since they rarely were consulted in the hospital's decision to discharge the patient. Social workers within family service agencies were similarly reluctant to deal with a discharged hospital patient, disliking the patient's pathology as well as the hospital psychiatrists' perceived aloofness and inaccessibility when needed. Effective relationships with new community resources were also constrained by the regulations and limited funds of the several other state agencies potentially capable of participating in the rehabilitation of discharged patients. Each of these public programs imposed unique requirements for the use of its resources, and considerable hospital effort had to be expended in satisfying these administrative demands.

The hospital was eminently more successful in quickly forging links for discharged patients with local nursing homes and visiting nurses, perhaps because of the staff's greater comfort and experience in working with medically oriented agencies. Although nursing homes had initially resisted accepting any psychiatric patients out of fear of repelling better behaved medical patients, this concern had been placated and over 600 chronic Boston State Hospital patients had been transferred to these facilities during the mid-1960s (Stotsky, 1966). In fact, most nursing homes no longer adhered to rigid quotas for psychiatric patients, and some senior psychiatrists urged that restrictions again be set lest the homes become mini–mental hospitals.

Links between the hospital and its catchment area generally developed on a decentralized basis, with community agency workers relating directly to the personnel of a specific hospital unit. Although this arrangement resulted in uneven hospital involvement with community resources, the linkages that were established worked effectively and served as potential models for all of the hospital's decentralized services. This pattern of decentralized hospital-community relationships was also appropriate, since no active and strong interagency council existed within the catchment area through which wide-ranging organizational relationships could be centrally and readily negotiated. The scattered social service and health resources located in the outlying areas of West Roxbury, Hyde Park and Roslindale generally were branches of major "downtown" Boston agencies, and they related more readily to the central parent organization than to the few neighboring facilities. An interagency council composed of almost two dozen health and social welfare resources did exist in Dorchester and had been instrumental several years earlier in pressing for a child guidance clinic. The council lay dormant, however, and the hospital's representative to it was a rehabilitation counselor rather than a member of the central administration.

Thus, Boston State Hospital clearly recognized the value of expanding its interactions and program linkages to psychiatric and nonpsychiatric resources which could share in the massive burden of treating the community's mentally ill. The opportunities for linkage expansion were constrained, however, by the hospital medical staff's personal inexperience and reluctance to initiate necessary community contacts, as well as by the hesitancy of many local agencies to assume new responsibilities for psychiatric patients. Successes had been achieved in some units as the result of direct, personalized efforts, but no clear procedures existed for generalizing hospital-community interaction patterns to all units of the psychiatric institution and to the several sectors in its catchment area.

THE NEIGHBORHOOD SERVICE CENTER

As a counterpoint to the various ambivalent efforts of hospital personnel to shift program emphases from institutional to community-based activities, it is instructive to consider the manner in which this goal was pursued by a hospital subsystem with a strong commitment to community mental health ideology (as measured by the 1967 Baker-Schulberg CMHI Scale). We had noted earlier that the hospital's home treatment service (Weiner, Becker, & Friedman, 1967) was unique in its ability to provide community-based clinical services and in its willingness to work closely with local medical and nonmedical caregivers. As a natural evolution of these well-established programs and in keeping with emerging emphases upon primary prevention, the director and some colleagues on the home treatment service focused their energies in 1966–1967 upon establishing a neighborhood service center (NSC). Creative, pioneering mental health programs are generated most effectively when complex organizational and environmental forces are properly harnessed in synchronous rather than incompatible ways. The rationale and strategies for establishing an NSC must, then, be considered in relation to the diverse national and local environmental forces affecting the hospital's development, while its specific programs must also be analyzed in the context of wide-ranging staff interests and reference groups, fluctuating funding opportunities, community and citizen priorities for services, and even fortuitous events.

The national climate at the time of the neighborhood service center's inception was a volatile one. Opposition to the Vietnam War was beginning to surface, and violent riots in many urban centers had pitted the nation's poor against the "establishment." Among the government's responses to such confrontations was the funding of numerous Office of Economic Opportunity antipoverty programs, upon the assumption that growing malaise could thereby be quelled. The Federal Community Mental Health Centers and Staffing Acts of 1963 and 1964, although conceived from humanitarian concerns predating these explosions, became an integral component of the nation's multiple quests to limit disturbances and move towards a "Great Society." The National Institute of Mental Health, as its contribution, assigned a high priority to grant applications addressing the mental health and social welfare needs of poor and minority populations.

The availability of substantial federal funds for community mental health services to treat the poor meshed perfectly with Boston State Hospital's desire to expand its programmatic base beyond institutional services. In fact, the hospital's superintendent at the time, Dr. Milton Greenblatt, had repeatedly encouraged staff to aggressively seek federal support for demonstration projects. A community mental health center staffing grant to establish a neighborhood service center was consistent with the superintendent's social psychiatric orientation; and he, therefore, encouraged this entrepreneurial activity because of the potential contribution to the hospital's overall development.

Given this highly supportive national and local environment, the director of the home treatment service turned his energy in 1966–1967 to drafting and refining an NIMH staffing grant application which sought to emulate the then highly acclaimed, ghetto-based Lincoln Hospital community mental health program in New York. The Boston State Hospital group subscribed in many ways to the problems-in-living rationale underlying the Lincoln Hospital program—i.e., the individual's maladjustment is not an entirely intrapsychic process but instead reflects a disequilibrium between the individual and his environment. This conceptual approach implies that psychotherapy with individuals produces only limited results. Lincoln Hospital staff espoused that professional's shift orientation and efforts accordingly "to understanding and changing whole segments of society [Peck, Roman, & Kaplan, 1967, p. 104]." Boston State Hospital staff similarly asserted that "it is our firm conviction that the responsibility of a community mental health center goes far beyond treatment of the mentally ill and that the center must make a major commitment to primary prevention, including collaboration with all other community resources in attacking the community's social ills that spawn continued social pathology and mental illness [Becker, Wylan, & McCourt, 1971, p. 412]."

The translation of this farreaching aspiration into definable, practical activities has plagued many well-intentioned mental health professionals, and similar travails were to be experienced by the group at Boston State Hospital. Feelings of citizen alientation and powerlessness as well as the invidious living conditions fostering them were deemed to be legitimate target problems by the NSC planners who were interested in developing programs of primary prevention. Nevertheless, the proposed range of services specified in the grant application reflected the staff's uncertainty as to whether the NSC was basically intended to ameliorate pathological social conditions affecting total populations (primary prevention), or to assist individuals with various forms of distress (secondary prevention). In consultation with the local antipoverty agency, the NSC staff initially designed a staffing grant application to fund a Lincoln Hospital-type storefront center on a major local thoroughfare. Among the services to be provided by it to the community were a "psychosocial first-aid station" offering screening and referral help; a therapeutic social club for such groups as the elderly, the socially isolated, and discharged patients; and a comprehensive alcoholism treatment program. To the outsider, the planned program seemed on balance directed more towards insuring accessible, relevant clinical services for psychiatrically and socially troubled individuals than towards tackling those factors affecting the quality of life and the social fabric of a rapidly changing community. In any event, the grant application was of sufficiently high quality and clearly addressed the needs of a minority, poverty population so that it was funded by NIMH.

While Boston State Hospital's administration negotiated legislative approval of the NIMH grant's state matching component so that the NSC could become operational by July 1968, NSC staff collected further data about the community's view of its major service needs. Extensive earlier contacts by the NSC's professional staff with community agencies, clergymen, general practitioners, etc., had made the hospital group aware of the many community needs addressed in the staffing grant. However, door-to-door interviews by newly recruited neighborhood mental health workers determined that local citizens perceived the lack of clubhouse-type services for young children, rather than clinical ones for adults, to be the community's most pressing problem.

This finding confronted the NSC planners with the need to choose between their own program interests and the community's expressed desires. At this critical juncture, a variety of fortuitous factors led the NSC personnel to conclude that although developing a clubhouse at which children could pursue constructive activities was markedly different in function and target population from the initial plan for an adult-oriented storefront center, the need was genuine and should be met. This decision was based on the facts that no funds had been provided in the staffing grant to rent storefront facilities; a recently emptied hospital building was available and accessible to the community; and a local neighborhood improvement association, with which the NSC had developed initial relationships, was interested in actively collaborating in establishing a community center. Furthermore, such a facility on the grounds of Boston State Hospital could help to break down suspiciousness between the hospital and its community; it would provide the staff with further opportunities to become familiar with neighborhood families and their needs. Within the relatively brief period of three months, the NSC's original purposes were drastically revamped, a tenuous working relationship was negotiated with the neighborhood improvement association, and state approval was obtained so that a community center could be opened on the hospital's grounds in July 1968.

The center flourished during the subsequent year, and Becker, Wylan, and McCourt (1971) reported that over 400 children participated during the 1969–1970 season in group programs, educational activities, medical-dental screening and housing project services. Many other preventive programs were subsequently developed including school intervention and consultation services, a family intervention unit, a children's developmental workshop, a residential treatment center, a children's day care center, a court program, a widows' program, a community consultation program, a community organization unit and an alcoholism prevention program.

The NSC's ability to function as an innovative, semiautonomous subsystem linking the hospital and community via preventive services must also be considered in relation to developments within the larger organization of which it was a part. As a result of the hospital's several phases of decentralization between 1967 and 1970, another semiautonomous clinical unit had been established to provide inpatient and outpatient clinical services to residents of the NSC's catchment area. By 1970, it became apparent to the clinical unit head and the hospital's central administration that separate specialized units were dysfunctional for both service as well as training purposes. A new structural approach for insuring integration and systemic unity, therefore, was necessary.

Merging a clinically oriented subsystem serving one geographic area with another clinical subsystem serving a neighboring area into a single mini-center can be easily decided upon; the organizational fate of a preventively oriented NSC is a more complex decision. The overall rationale of the hospital's several reorganization plans, i.e., providing comprehensive services and continuity of care to the catchment area, favored integration of the NSC into the new minicenter. However, legitimate concerns were expressed that the NSC's loss of autonomy would submerge preventive goals in favor of ever-pressing clinical needs. The initial decision, therefore, was to maintain the "mission integrity" of the NSC. Inevitable problems continued, though, in providing comprehensive services to the community. Linkages between the NSC and the hospital's clinically oriented mini-center were hard to establish, overlapping community efforts combining clinical and preventive features were difficult to coordinate and mutual blaming was common (Sharaf, Kaplan, & Cole, 1971). The NSC's separate status was deemed sufficiently dysfunctional to the hospital's overall purposes that in the late winter of 1971 it was reorganized as a component of the related mini-center, a merger simplified by the fact that the NSC's director was away then on educational leave. As Sharaf, Kaplan, & Cole have suggested, it remains to be seen whether the preventive services launched earlier by the NSC can continue to develop and flourish in the absence of a shielding, semiautonomous administrative structure.

This brief description of the NSC's gestation, rapid growth and subsequent merger into a larger hospital system highlights the fact that such programs develop and function within the context of various organizationally and temporally meshing elements. Using our model of organizational groupings as "people— belief— resource" systems, it is clear that the NSC's initial activities stemmed from the ability of key staff members subscribing to community mental health ideology within a receptive environment to obtain federal and state funds. The absence of any of these elements could have aborted the NSC's birth and development.

Finally, it is also clear that a subsystem which grows at a disproportionately rapid rate generates intolerable tensions within the larger system of which it is a component. The NSC's proliferating community programs and extensive environmental linkages created an imbalance vis-à-vis the hospital's clinical units and threatened the institution's integrative capacity, an intolerable situation which the administration resolved by merging the involved components. It, thus, is obvious that a subsystem's plans for community-oriented services cannot develop in isolation from the parent organization's requirements and priorities. In fact, inordinate success when proceeding on a semiautonomous basis may actually contribute to the subsystem's demise, a paradox noted by Etzioni (1960) in his analysis of the goal-attainment model's limitations for program evaluation.

SUMMARY

This chapter has briefly reviewed some of the many community systems with which the mental hospital interacts in its quest to achieve new goals, and the concepts of open-systems theory have been used as an integrative thread. One cannot help but be impressed, and perhaps even overwhelmed, by the range of activity which the hospital must sustain if it is to achieve its goals of effective patient care, training and research. The hospital constantly is being challenged to shed its traditional provincial self-concept and to adopt a broad-ranging community-oriented perspective through which it can assume a position of strength in negotiating future roles. Whether the mental hospital's personnel, the vast majority of whom have been trained to gaze inward, can now turn equal attention to the myriad of environmental forces by which they are surrounded represents the greatest challenge to the growth of hospital-community linkages.

We would be remiss, however, if we failed to emphasize that in addition to the many successful linkages which can be developed, there exist also situations of friction. A frequent result of increased organizational interaction is not only cooperation but also competitiveness and conflict. As the mental hospital's role evolves, it may become engaged in disputes with other resources over fiscal allocations, personnel and even domain prerogatives. These will not be easy matters to resolve, but a favorable climate for seeking a solution will be created if the mental hospital remembers that just as it possesses a body of expertise which it offers to its caregiving colleagues, so do other resources possess valuable skills which they are willing to share with the hospital. We also would suggest that in addition to traditional reciprocal consultative arrangements with medical-type facilities, new ones be developed with such resources as group work agencies, community caregivers, lawyers and environmental analysts. Such steps will facilitate the ultimate definition of a "community" and the optimal structure of its mental health system.

10. *Clinical Programs and Patient Outcome*

The study of organizational change within the framework of open systems concepts involves the analysis of many general and specific functions which the focal organization strives to fulfill in its quest for viability and relevance. The analysis must recognize that organizations are dynamic. Their functions shift because of fluctuating environmental demands, the varying availability of needed resources and changing system goals. In the preceding chapters we have considered the issues confronting a traditionally oriented mental hospital seeking contemporary clinical, training and research functions consistent with the community mental health role sanctioned for it by the state legislature. These changes were related to a changing ideological climate affecting system goals, evolving decentralized structures designed to maintain subsystem integration and coordination in the face of strong internal and external pressures towards differentiation, and modified professional roles and relationships for better meeting the needs of those seeking direct and indirect services from the hospital's several subsystems. Within this broad framework, the changing mental hospital was shown to meet the parameters of an open "people—belief—resource" (PBR) system as described in Chapter 4.

PBR systems of the human services type follow a basic cyclic character and have activity patterns similar to those of other organizational systems. They accept inputs from the environment, transform these inputs via technologies organized into throughput subsystems, and return outputs to the environment. The major inputs to a mental hospital were defined in Chapter 4 as patients, staff and students, legitimation, technology and material; the key throughput structures were identified as the patient-care, training, research, boundary-spanning and managerial and administrative subsystems; and the outputs were specified as including discharged patients, trained or educated personnel, research reports, change in level of health among the community's population, patient maintenance programs and community education.

It is clear from the perspective of the open systems model that organizational change can be appropriately analyzed along any or all of these input-throughput-output dimensions. This chapter will limit itself, however, to examining the mental hospital's "people-processing" activities, i.e., the nature of patient-care programs provided by a community mental health–oriented institution. Particular emphasis will be placed upon the changing characteristics of those people seeking care and the clinical structures and procedures through which a mental hospital accepts human inputs; the clinical practices or treatment technologies whereby the mental hospital processes individuals through its inpatient subsystems; and the nature of organizational outputs as reflected in the outcome for cohorts of patients treated by the mental hospital at different points in time. This input-throughput-output analysis, which expands upon the evaluative model initially presented in Chapter 6 in relation to the effects of unitization, perforce remains more paradigmatic than comprehensive. Difficulties in obtaining necessary organizational data, limited research personnel and time constraints precluded as thorough a data-gathering program as our conceptual framework dictates. Nevertheless, the following open systems analysis of patient flow through the mental hospital is still relatively unique, and this chapter is deemed significant for its modelbuilding implications as well as for the data which it presents.

THE MENTAL HOSPITAL'S HUMAN INPUTS

The functioning and effectiveness of any "people-belief-resource" system such as a mental hospital is very much dependent upon the characteristics of the clients whom it processes, i.e., age, sex, diagnosis and the other variables which abet or limit staff's therapeutic success. The hospital's acceptance and treatment of new human inputs is also constrained by the needs of individuals for whom the organization already is clinically responsible, as well as by the potential demands of a broader range of community residents seeking benefits from the hospital's services. Thus, the mental hospital's ability to accept, let alone expand, inputs so as to include those relevant to community mental health goals is a complex process.

One of the most severe constraints upon most hospitals' ability to easily accept, effectively treat and rapidly discharge new patients is the backlog of chronic cases upon whom even limited organizational resources must be expended. We have reviewed in earlier chapters the managerial and clinical problems associated with hard-core populations, and the urgency of reducing their numbers so that scarce personnel can be freed for work with new types of community needs. An analysis of the composition of Boston State Hospital's clientele when our study began in 1965–1966 revealed that 62 percent of those in treatment were the responsibility of inpatient subsystems (Table 10-1); the vast majority of these inpatients were decidedly chronic as well as elderly.

Table 10-1
Boston State Hospital's Patient Population 1965–1966

Unit	*No.*	*Median Age*	*Median Months Since Most Recent Admission*
Inpatient	1,880	57.6	80.4
Drug Addiction Clinic	78	44.6	5.4
Family Care	82	53.4	13.9
Day Care	134	39.4	7.9
Aftercare	501	55.4	10.7
Geriatric Aftercare	96	60+	9.2
Outpatient Clinic	131	32.5	10.7
Home Treatment	143	43.4	10.2
	3,045		

The processes which produced silting patterns, i.e., a growing backlog of chronic patients, at Boston State Hospital (Kantor & Gelineau, 1969; Kris, Schiff, & McLaughlin, 1971) were typical of those prevalent at other large psychiatric institutions. Kantor and Gelineau concluded that the social processes and structures of a typical Boston State Hospital chronic ward had not only failed to be therapeutic but were *antitherapeutic* in spite of the therapeutic ideology more or less accepted by front-line staff. The sizable component of geriatric individuals resident at Boston State Hospital in 1965 (46 percent of the total inpatient census) similarly stemmed from nontherapeutic factors long at play within most psychiatric institutions and their surrounding environments (Hefferin & Wilner, 1971; Stotsky, 1972).

Nevertheless, it is clear that, despite a variety of lingering staff resistances to organizational change, Boston State Hospital has significantly reduced the size of its overwhelming inpatient population, particularly the backlog of chronically ill individuals. During the decade of the 1960s the inpatient census was reduced 66 percent in the face of a relatively stable admissions pattern (Table 10-2). Perhaps most remarkable is that in contrast to widespread predictions that census decreases would level off as the "easier" patients are discharged, the fact is that Boston State Hospital accelerated its inpatient reduction during the latter half of the decade. Annual census decreases averaged 6 percent from 1960 to 1965, but jumped to 14 percent annually from 1965 to 1970. Between October 1963 and October 1968 the segment of the inpatient population which had been hospitalized for at least five straight years dropped from 61 percent to 44 percent of the total group. Thus, the numerous programmatic endeavors described in earlier chapters, and by Greenblatt, Sharaf, & Stone (1971), were instrumental in profoundly altering the organizational context

Table 10-2
Boston State Hospital Inpatients

	Admissions		Resident Census	
Year	*No.*	*% Change*	*No.*	*% Change*
1960	2018		2669	
1961	1805	−10.5	2465	− 7.8
1962	1762	− 2.4	2322	− 5.8
1963	1894	7.5	2298	− 1.3
1964	1917	1.2	2154	− 6.3
1965	2003	4.5	1956	− 8.9
1966	1885	− 5.9	1610	−17.6
1967	1945	3.2	1349	−16.1
1968	1756	− 9.7	1218	−10.1
1969	1734	− 1.3	1043	−14.4
1970	1725	− 0.5	895	−14.2

into which Boston State Hospital accepted patient inputs as it expanded community mental health activities. In fact, a patient census in late 1968 of the hospital's various subsystems revealed that the segment being treated through inpatient units had dropped from 62 percent in 1965 to 50 percent in 1968; conversely, the segment of individuals under the care of outpatient and community-based subsystems had grown from 38 percent to 50 percent of the hospital's total during this same period.

Having noted the changing organizational emphases and the diminishing constraints on processing newly admitted patients, we now will describe "people" inputs to Boston State Hospital during our study's time-frame. A fundamental principle of community mental health theory is that of focusing upon populations rather than identified patients alone; i.e., the mental health professional accepts responsibility for not only those patients who seek his help but also for the unidentified, potentially ill members of his community. However, to the staff of a mental hospital which for years has been overwhelmed by the diverse clinical needs of countless individuals seeking its services, active casefinding for additional unidentified clients often is a task of the lowest priority. The more relevant issue becomes that of how the institution can expand its scope of responsibility and provide services to at least those clients whom it had previously rejected, e.g., alcoholic or violent individuals. At Boston State Hospital, many staff recognized that if their facility aspired to function as a community mental health center, they could not continue to routinely exclude difficult patients. A wide gap existed, however, between the positive inclinations of administrative staff to adopt a broader intake policy and the reluctance of clinical staff to assume the practical responsibilities related to the care of troublesome individuals.

Resolving the mental hospital's legitimate scope of responsibility in community mental health programs is also hampered by the ambiguity of whether related services will be available from local human services organizations. For example, if the mental hospital provides inpatient detoxification to alcoholics, can these individuals obtain community services such as vocational rehabilitation when indicated? There is little question that a mental hospital aspiring to the title of "community mental health center" is responsible for treating alcoholics and other previously excluded client groups. However, staff reluctance to undertake strange tasks, as well as lingering concerns about the extent of cooperation available from other community caregivers, remain to be resolved before many hospitals will effectively expand their scope of clinical responsibility.

The manner in which Boston State Hospital's inputs changed in accordance with its growing community mental health orientation can be viewed through an analysis of the cohort of individuals admitted from the Dorchester neighborhood of its catchment area during the first six months of 1967. The policy and orientation of the various hospital subsystems through which people are admitted for care are particularly relevant to an input analysis. Prior to 1967 the physician in Boston State Hospital's admissions office felt himself to have the choice of admitting an individual to an inpatient ward, or refusing him treatment. Since most residents selected the more clinically conservative alternative, the inpatient subsystem was the hospital's primary vehicle for responding to those seeking help. Recognizing the problems that were thus created in terms of chronicity and difficulty in returning the individual to his community, many staff members urged that inpatient admissions be reduced and other options developed. The superintendent even expressed the hope that procedures ultimately could be devised for screening all patients in the community so that they wouldn't even have to come to the hospital. As an initial step towards developing an expanded range of treatment subsystems, the outpatient clinic dropped its longstanding practice of excluding most non-neurotic individuals. Team screening was subsequently undertaken by the clinic staff members, and they particularly strived to design nonresidential treatment plans for the sizable group of alcoholics and chronic schizophrenics who usually are admitted to mental hospitals in the absence of community alternatives.

Given Boston State Hospital's goal of expanding community-based care, it therefore was not surprising to find in our study of the 1967 cohort that 49 percent of the Dorchester residents contacting the institution were accepted for care by the outpatient clinics and the home treatment service, while 51 percent were admitted to inpatient subsystems. Of the latter group requiring 24-hour care, approximately 60 percent went directly to the newly established unit responsible for their geographic area, another 35 percent were admitted to the hospital's medical, geriatric and screening specialty units, while the remaining 5 percent were assigned to other inpatient units for administrative reasons. Thus, during the initial half of 1967, Boston State Hospital's nonresidential subsystems accepted as many people inputs from its catchment area as did the organization's residential subsystems—a reasonable ratio for a psychiatric organization whose traditional emphasis had been upon inpatient care.

A less sanguine feature of Boston State Hospital's programmatic transition was the fact that virtually no partial hospitalization subsystems existed in 1967 as a further clinical alternative in the input decisionmaking process. Despite a variety of findings about the efficacy of this treatment option (e.g. Zwerling & Wilder, 1964; Wilder,

Levin, & Zwerling, 1966), Boston State Hospital was unable to elaborate this type of caregiving subsystem so as to avoid the inpatient admission of seriously ill individuals. Partial hospitalization remains relatively underutilized and unrefined in many other psychiatric institutions as well (Glasscote et al., 1969; Gross, 1971) even though it is deemed one of the five essential community mental health services. The reasons may stem from staff and community's unfamiliarity with the service's theoretic rationale, staff and families' reluctance to hazard questionable clinical decisions and perhaps even staff's hesitancy to elaborate another treatment subsystem with which clinical decisions and program resources will have to be shared.

In addition to determining the expanded subsystem entry points to the changing mental hospital, it is meaningful to analyze whether type of subsystem utilization is related to client or community characteristics. A study of Boston State Hospital's 1967 cohort revealed that the pattern whereby Dorchester residents were accepted to the hospital's inpatient and outpatient subsystems varied considerably; in fact, the rank order correlation between the inpatient and outpatient utilization rates for the area's 34 census tracts was only .02. Significantly more inpatients than outpatients were admitted to the hospital from census tracts located in the North Dorchester neighborhoods with poor, predominantly black populations. Equal utilization rates of inpatient and outpatient subsystems were found among the residents of census tracts fairly adjacent to the hospital's physical location. Significantly higher numbers of individuals were admitted to the hospital's outpatient rather than inpatient subsystems from the relatively stable, predominantly white Irish census tracts in South Dorchester. Additional variables on which the total Dorchester outpatient and inpatient cohorts varied are those of age and marital status—characteristics long associated with differing prognoses and treatment approaches. Only 7 percent of those accepted for outpatient care were 60 years of age and older while 21 percent of the inpatient group were in the geriatric group. Similarly, 54 percent of the outpatients were married while only 36 percent of those admitted for 24-hour care had spouses.

Yuchtman & Seashore (1967) have suggested that organizational change may be appropriately assessed in terms of modified inputs and input subsystems as well as on the conventional criteria of outputs. The inputs to a "people-belief-resource" organizational system such as a mental hospital have been described as the community residents who seek professional care—a service which traditionally was undertaken by admitting the applicant to an inpatient subsystem. Our earlier analysis of Boston State Hospital's changing ideology and program goals was now shown to be operationally related to modified input procedures. As a consequence, a growing number of individuals were being accepted for treatment through nonresidential subsystems. Although the patterns of outpatient and inpatient care still varied with a person's age, race and marital status, Boston State Hospital's clientele and input subsystems increasingly were assuming community mental health characteristics and moving away from the delimited concerns of traditional mental hospitals.

THE MENTAL HOSPITAL'S TREATMENT TECHNOLOGIES

The relevance and efficiency of an organization's throughput procedures determine its ability to convert the inputs which it receives from the environment into appropriate outputs. The mental hospital functioning as a community mental health center must organize its treatment subsystems so as to maximize therapeutic rather than custodial technologies. Greenblatt (1972) has described the evolution of mental hospital throughput procedures as passing through several historic phases: the custodial authoritarian period of the 1920s and 1930s; the therapeutic egalitarian era of the 1950s; the comprehensive community mental health center period of the late 1960s; and the total health care model of the future. The metamorphosis, Greenblatt emphasizes, has resulted from a complex mosaic of movement and interchanges between the hospital and society based upon deeply meaningful and powerfully motivated concerns.

Although the role of society's legislators and citizens in the development of treatment models has been well recognized, the evolution towards therapeutic technologies is also being greatly stimulated by a series of legal actions (Burris, 1969). A series of judicial decrees starting with the 1966 District Court of Columbia decision in *Rouse* v. *Cameron* have held that committed mental patients have the right to treatment and that mental hospitals must organize and provide appropriate therapies. The failure to provide treatment raises constitutional questions of due process, equal protection and cruel and unusual punishment.

The 1971 decision and the 1972 judicial order of the Alabama Federal District Court in *Wyatt* v. *Stickney* reiterated the constitutional guarantee of the right to treatment, and defined three programmatic areas basic to the fulfillment of this right: (1) a humane psychological and physical environment; (2) qualified staff in numbers sufficient to administer adequate treatment; and (3) individualized treatment plans. Ironically, widespread application of the Alabama judicial order requiring significant expenditures for services *within* institutions may well preclude expansion of community-based services because of the limited funds available within any state for mental health programs (Kaplan, 1973).

Nevertheless, it is evident that despite the potential for systemic paradoxes and programmatic imbalances, treatment procedures within psychiatric organizations are now subject to not only professional judgment but judicial scrutiny as well. As efforts to implement professional and judicial requirements continue, the lack of objective treatment standards becomes all the more troublesome. For example, lawyers deem the American Psychiatric Association's "Standards For Psychiatric Facilities" (1969) inadequate since they omit mandatory staff-patient ratios. Psychiatrists, on the other hand, consider such ratios to be potentially harmful, since they can function as maximal rather than minimal indices of needed personnel.

Professionals are aware of the ambiguous approaches pursued by psychiatric organizations in delivering treatment services, and recent studies (e.g., Ullmann, 1967; Linn, 1970; Ellsworth & Maroney, 1972; and Goldstein et al. 1972) have sought to clarify the variables associated with optimal clinical functioning. Hospital size and staffing ratios consistently emerge as crucial organizational factors affecting patient outcome. Using rapid patient discharge as a criterion of effectiveness, Ullmann (1967) found in a study of 30 Veterans Administration neuropsychiatric facilities that: (1) as hospital size increases, hospital effectiveness decreases; (2) an increased number of staff members per patient is positively associated with greater effectiveness because staff-patient contact increases; and (3) smaller hospitals have greater staff participation and, therefore, are more effective.

In juxtaposition to the lingering ambivalences and resistances of many mental hospitals about contemporary treatment technologies, other facilities have moved to implement faddish "prestige" treatment packages. The package's contents in the San Francisco area include an open-door policy, a permissive approach to the patient, a team approach to decisions, a degree of patient government, and no electroconvulsive therapy (Fischer & Weinstein, 1971). Each of these treatment elements may be desirable in its own right, but Fischer & Weinstein are concerned that psychiatric facilities, in their search for enlightenment, are slavishly adopting the prestige package in its entirety. During the 1960s, adherents of the psychotherapeutic, somatotherapeutic, and sociotherapeutic orientations (Armor & Klerman, 1968) stressed the unique and exclusive virtues of their particular approaches. The result was a loss in the diversity and flexibility needed to give optimal treatment to varied patient populations. This problem will continue so long as the etiology of mental illness remains unresolved and treatment programs are based upon changing orientations. The manner in which the interrelated variables of changing ideological orientation, treatment technology and organizational structure affect patient care can be seen in the following review of Boston State Hospital's efforts to modify throughput procedures in accordance with its growing role as a community mental health center.

The 1965–1970 period of our study was one of profound change in Boston State Hospital's clinical and treatment activities. The previously prestigious psychoanalytic concepts and techniques embodied in the psychotherapeutic orientation, and utilized primarily on inpatient services, diminished in centrality. The superintendents displayed an affinity for eclectic approaches, and community-oriented rather than hospital-based activities assumed a significantly higher priority. The merits of the therapeutic milieu generated fresh interest among staff, and many ward administrators established treatment programs loosely rooted in these concepts. Day-care programs were increasingly utilized, and some staff even advocated that patients not be admitted to the institution unless family members participated in the admission workup.

An institution's movement away from existing treatment orientations often is not a smooth one. Instead, it may be marked by continuing controversy over clinical and administrative issues whose ultimate resolution profoundly affects the structure and effectiveness of community mental health services. At Boston State Hospital, the psychoanalytically trained staff opposed many of the new clinical directions, and they voiced a concern that was to echo through the institution for several years. They contended that patient care was being deleteriously affected by staff ineptly utilizing social-psychiatric techniques, and that patients were suffering from the superficial care provided by those whose primary interest was in discharging patients back to the community. In fact, they asserted, patients were not even obtaining a basic admission workup with its inherent therapeutic potential. Psychoanalytically oriented staff were also deeply concerned about the hospital's increased difficulty in recruiting personnel to work on inpatient services, since many young professionals chose assignments on the supposedly relevant and glamorous community-based services. To the psychoanalytically oriented staff, this job preference was but further evidence of the mental health professional's growing inability to sustain the intimacy and commitment required to treat longterm or severely disturbed patients.

In addition to the basic differences evident among staff in a changing mental hospital regarding choice of clinical technologies, differences also arise between key personnel about the optimal organizational structures and administrative practices relevant to community mental health pursuits. For example, many staff anticipate that an expanded array of services will assure the patient continuity of care through the various phases of his illness. At Boston State Hospital, the geographically based unit system was viewed as the organizational structure for achieving this goal, since patients always would be treated by their community's unit. However, an overly rigid adherence to this policy could be detrimental if the semiautonomous units refused to treat former patients who do not reside within the newly established catchment area boundaries. Would the previously established goal of an ever-decreasing patient census, or the newly accepted one of continuity of care for all patients, be the more important goal for the unit to achieve?

The complexity of instituting continuity of care as a key throughput procedure can also be seen in the fact that at Boston State Hospital most ward psychiatrists didn't give their patients physical examinations, since this ran counter to the psychoanalytic treatment model; a significant number of patients were transferred annually to general hospitals for medical consultations and procedures. Within a year after first establishing the unit system, the hospital adopted the policy of having the unit psychiatrist who would be responsible for the patient administer the examination, rather than having it performed by admitting room personnel. Opposition to this clinical practice, nevertheless, was to linger for some time.

Although the several phases of Boston State Hospital's unitization (described in Chapter 6) successively eliminated obstacles to new clinical procedures, the goal of comprehensive services and continuity of care remained only partially fulfilled as long as the pressures for organizational differentiation and integration competed with each other. The freedom provided decentralized units to experiment with unique treatment approaches was significant in attracting new staff and boosting morale, but comprehensive services could not be achieved unless independent ventures were integrated into the hospital's total organizational structure.

Another complex decision associated with changing technological procedures and priorities in the changing mental hospital is the degree to which staff will commit itself to active treatment of the hundreds of chronic patients already residing within the institution. Disproportionately greater resources generally are assigned to the treatment of acute, newly admitted patients, while long-term patients traditionally receive custodial care from the few personnel assigned to their wards. At Boston State Hospital, establishment of the unit system brought this issue into sharper focus and forced fresh decisions about the numbers and types of personnel to be distributed among chronic and acute patient clinical programs. Equitably staffed teams responsible for the care of both types of patients could be developed so that the active therapeutic modalities employed with acutely ill individuals would also be directed toward the chronic ones; conversely, teams of differing sizes could be maintained in keeping with staff predilections and the traditionally differing clinical approaches to the needs of the two patient groups. Both staffing patterns are problematic—the former since the plan of a single team providing active treatment for both acute and chronic patients might be nothing more than a fantasy, and the latter since it would perpetuate the existing clinical pattern which discriminates against chronic patients.

Treatment Surveys

Longitudinal analyses of the clinical technologies utilized by hospital staff in treating patients can reveal the direction and magnitude of evolving organizational activities. Although few treatment surveys have been reported in the psychiatric literature, they constitute a sensitive barometer of shifting institutional environments and provide a framework within which mental hospitals can assess their emerging treatment efforts. Such surveys are particularly valuable in helping to determine the relationship between management-level goals and the daily staff activities being utilized for their implementation.

The overt thrust of Boston State Hospital's activities and services during the decade of the 1960s was in the direction of intensified, organizationwide therapeutic care for all patients. The principles of community mental health ideology had achieved growing prominence, administrative changes such as the unit system were being implemented and the reduced inpatient census had significantly improved staff-patient ratios. Although impressive at the global, organizational level of analysis, were these presumably positive thrusts indeed producing individualized care for all patients? We sought to clarify this fundamental question through a series of treatment surveys designed to indicate: (1) the ways in which a changing mental hospital deploys its treatment resources, and (2) the relationship of patients' characteristics to their participation in treatment.

In the falls of 1965 and 1968, the authors and their colleagues conducted inpatient treatment surveys at Boston State Hospital (Schulberg, Notman, & Bookin, 1967; Schulberg & Wojcik, 1971). Each study was of the point-prevalence type, so that we first obtained the names of all in-patients living in the hospital on the dates of our surveys. We then determined from each staff member the names of every inpatient being treated by him on these dates. For purposes of our study, a patient was defined as being in treatment with a staff member if work was started before the survey date and the staff member considered that "there is a definite and continuing commitment for further work" with this patient. This definition was specifically intended to exclude from our study the many patients with whom a psychiatrist has only an administrative relationship, and the random treatment provided by staff through ward group activity programs in which there is no commitment made to develop a treatment relationship with a specific individual patient.

Each staff member was asked to provide on a data form the names of all patients he was treating and the category of treatment received by each patient. The categories as specified on the forms included variations of verbal therapy (e.g., individual and group psychotherapy, counseling and casework) and variations of activity treatment (e.g., industrial and occupational therapy). A staff member's designation of the type of treatment being provided to a patient was accepted at face value, since in a hospitalwide study we could not check into the finer subtleties of whether, for example, a patient was in fact receiving psychotherapy or counseling. Data on current drug treatment were provided from patients' charts by the nursing staff of every ward in the hospital. Since electric shock treatments were administered in a central unit, the names of all patients receiving this other form of somatic therapy also could be determined accurately. Behavioral therapy had not yet been initiated by hospital staff (even at the time of our last survey in 1968), and no information about this technology's utilization is included in this report.

The data forms distributed to hospital staff members at the time of each survey were returned within three months by every member of the psychiatry, psychology, social service, rehabilitation, occupational therapy, volunteer and chaplain services. Nursing was the only service from which complete information could not be obtained in each of the surveys. Only 57 percent of the nursing staff returned data forms in 1965, and 62 percent did so in 1968. However, most of the nonrespondents were attendants on the evening and night shifts, and we assumed that little specific treatment was provided during these hours. In view of the very high overall staff response rates to each of the surveys, the following data are deemed to be a comprehensive indication of inpatient treatment programs at the times of the studies.

The varying combinations of treatment provided to inpatients in 1963, 1965 and 1968 are shown in Table 10-3. The most significant finding is that the hospital's changing programs and increased emphasis upon direct patient services had reduced the number of patients receiving no specific treatment from 37 percent in 1963 to 13 percent in 1968. This reduction was primarily a result of the growing use of somatic therapies, prin-

Table 10-3
Percentage of Inpatients Receiving Various Types of Therapies in 1963, 1965, and 1968

	*1963**	*1965*	*1968*
Nothing specific	37	18	13
Verbal alone	4	5	3
Activity alone	11	6	2
Somatic alone	24	34	46
Verbal and activity	3	3	2
Verbal and somatic	4	11	16
Somatic and activity	10	14	9
Verbal, activity and somatic	7	9	9
Any verbal	18	28	30
Any activity	31	32	22
Any somatic	45	69	80

*Based upon data assembled by Dr. Ralph Notman, Boston University School of Medicine.

cipally medication, during this five-year period. Only 45 percent of the hospital's total population received somatic therapies in 1963, but by 1968 four out of every five inpatients were being treated in this way.

The verbal therapies had traditionally been regarded as the prestigious treatment of choice by Boston State Hospital's senior psychiatric staff. Indeed, the 1965 treatment survey had found a 50 percent increase since 1963 in the number of patients receiving this clinical service. However, by 1968 the proportion had increased only 2 percent and had stabilized at 30 percent of the hospital's total population. In point of fact, since the number of inpatients had dropped from 2,250 in October 1963 to 1,230 in October 1968, the actual number of inpatients receiving verbal therapies *decreased* over this time span despite a markedly improved staff-patient ratio. The decrease in verbal therapies was particularly sharp for group psychotherapy. In 1965 a total of 228 patients participated in groups, but the number had dropped to only 61 by 1968.

A significant component of the community mental health orientation espoused by the hospital's superintendent in the mid-1960s was the rehabilitation therapies designed to improve a patient's capacity for coping with life's daily tasks. Almost half of the hospital's inpatients had spent more than five years within the institution since their most recent admission, and their return to community living very much depended upon the acquisition of new functional skills. Data from the treatment surveys revealed that the various activity therapies expanded rapidly in the first part of the 1960s, but between 1965 and 1968 the percentage of patients involved in these clinical services decreased from 32 percent to only 22 percent of the total inpatient population. Again, this reduction is even more marked when considered in the light of the hospital's census drop from 1,880 to 1,230 inpatients between 1965 and 1968.

In view of the changing and flexible job descriptions deemed appropriate for mental health professionals in the context of community mental health ideology, the treatment surveys obtained data on the types of therapies provided patients by Boston State Hospital's various professional disciplines. We found in both 1965 and 1968 that psychiatrists, psychologists, social workers and clergymen engaged almost exclusively in verbal therapy—individual and group casework, counseling and psychotherapy. As might also be expected, rehabilitation and occupational therapy staff related to patients primarily through activity therapies. The nursing staff, which the earlier surveys had found to utilize almost every treatment modality, by 1968 was emphasizing verbal interactions of the individual counseling type—a development perhaps linked to this discipline's quest for greater prestige and power vis-à-vis professional colleagues.

We had noted earlier that an issue of major concern to the changing mental hospital emphasizing therapeutic rather than custodial care, is the question of whether to distribute scarce treatment resources equitably among the diverse patient populations, or to utilize resources selectively. This issue was a particularly crucial one at Boston State Hospital, where adoption of the unit system in 1966 was strongly motivated by staff's desire to equalize clinical services for all patients. Was the goal of active treatment on all units achieved?

Table 10-4 indicates that between 1965 and 1968 interunit variation in providing somatic treatments had been reduced. By 1968, between 75 and 90 percent of the patients on each unit were receiving drugs (the 1968 figures for somatic treatment refer almost exclusively to medications as only five of the 1,230 inpatients were receiving electroconvulsive therapy). The unit that showed the biggest change in treatment pattern was the

Table 10-4
Percentage of Patients in Various Hospital Units
Receiving Treatment in 1965 and 1968

	Any verbal	*Any activity*	*Any somatic*	*Nothing specific*
May unit				
1965 (N=167)	40	46	83	9
1968 (N=133)	53	27	90	2
Austin unit				
1965 (N=126)	77	36	81	4
1968 (N=99)	46	51	85	4
H-Complex				
1965 (N=617)	16	43	70	17
1968 (N=375)	21	31	79	13
Dorchester unit				
1965 (N=359)	40	36	77	9
1968 (N=110)	35	38	88	7
Geriatric unit				
1965 (N=366)	23	11	38	44
1968 (N=291)	23	5	75	19
Medical unit				
1965 (N=245)	11	3	83	14
1968 (N=199)	29	5	81	15

geriatric service, which in 1965 had been providing specific treatment to only 56 percent of its patients. Three years later, 81 percent were receiving specific treatment. The increase stemmed from the fact that the proportion of geriatric patients receiving drugs had nearly doubled in the interim—from 38 percent in 1965 to 75 percent in 1968.

The 1968 study continued to show distinct differences in the amounts of verbal therapy being provided by the several units. For instance, 53 percent of the patients on the May unit were taking part in some form of verbal therapy, as compared with 21 percent on the H-Complex. The Austin unit, which in 1965 had been the most active provider of verbal therapies, had reduced those services by 1968; the percentage of patients involved in such treatment had dropped from 77 to 46.

The distribution of activity therapy varied the most between treatment subsystems after the hospital's unitization. In 1965 about 40 percent of the patients on each of the four psychiatric units had been involved in such therapy, with a minimum of 36 percent and a maximum of 46 percent. In 1968 the range extended from 27 percent to 51 percent. Only 5 percent of the patients in the medical and geriatric units were receiving activity therapy at this latter time.

In addition to the question of whether an organization is deploying its resources more uniformly as the result of a modified administrative structure, our open systems analysis posed the question of whether the reorganized subsystems could increase the use of all relevant clinical technologies. Our findings at Boston State Hospital showed that all the reorganized units had indeed extended the use of two treatment modalities, but simultaneously reduced the use of a third (Table 10-4). Somatic and verbal therapies were now being used more extensively on the H-Complex and the May unit, but the proportion of patients in activity therapy had decreased. In the Dorchester and Austin units, somatic and activity therapies were more widespread in 1968 after unitization, but fewer patients received verbal therapies.

We had suggested earlier that decisions about the provision of clinical treatment are complex ones affected by organizational, technological and patient variables. In studying the pattern of how therapeutic care was distributed at Boston State Hospital, we sought to clarify

Table 10-5
Percentage of Inpatients Receiving Treatment in 1965 and 1968 by Age

	Any verbal	*Any activity*	*Any somatic*	*Nothing specific*
15–24 years				
1965 (N=84)	62	52	71	12
1968 (N=98)	59	49	77	12
25–39 years				
1965 (N=282)	45	44	85	7
1968 (N=200)	43	37	85	8
40–59 years				
1965 (N=652)	27	43	79	9
1968 (N=366)	27	28	82	10
60 and over				
1965 (N=860)	19	13	55	31
1968 (N=549)	22	9	77	7

whether a patient's personal characteristics were related to the type of treatment he received. In both the 1965 and 1968 treatment surveys, we found that age and length of time since the most recent admission were crucial variables. As Table 10-5 shows, a patient's participation in verbal therapy is directly related to his age. Approximately three out of five patients between the ages of 15 and 24 were involved in verbal therapy at the time of both the 1965 and 1968 studies; only one in five patients over 60 received such treatment. Moreover, although activity therapy was evenly distributed in 1965 among patients ranging in age from 15 to 59, the percentage of those over age 40 who were involved in such care in 1968 was sharply reduced. Few geriatric patients received activity therapy in either 1965 or 1968.

Table 10-5 also shows that the hospital's increased use of drugs occurred primarily with the geriatric group. Drug treatment among patients aged 15 to 59 remained stable between 1965 and 1968. However, the proportion of patients over age 60 being treated with drugs had increased from 55 percent to 77 percent by 1968. Thus, our study demonstrated a sharp reduction in the number of older patients not receiving any specific treatment, and their participation in at least one therapy was equal in 1968 to that of other age groups.

When Boston State Hospital adopted the unit system in 1966, the chronically ill patients housed on continued treatment services were redistributed among all of the new psychiatric units. The rationale for this change was that level of care could thereby be improved and that the longterm patients would no longer be isolated from active treatment programs. Did this in fact occur?

Table 10-6 indicates that at the time of the 1968 treatment survey there was, indeed, a reduction in the number of chronic patients not receiving at least one specific therapy. Again, this change seemed to be a result of the increased use of drugs in all phases of hospitalization. The use of verbal therapy with patients hospitalized less than two years was found increased between 1965 and 1968, but both surveys revealed that participation in such therapy declines as the patient's inpatient stay lengthens. The hospital's overall reduced level of activity therapy shown in Table 10-3 affected all patient groups regardless of length of stay. Whereas the 1965 survey found intensified activity services being offered to patients who had been in the hospital for more than ten years, the 1968 survey data did not reveal such staff efforts.

Table 10-6
Percentage of Inpatients Receiving Treatment
in 1965 and 1968 by Time Since Most Recent Admission

Length of stay	*Any verbal*	*Any activity*	*Any somatic*	*Nothing specific*
Less than two years				
1965 (N=546)	34	29	75	15
1968 (N=482)	40	21	82	11
Two to 10 years				
1965 (N=553)	34	27	67	21
1968 (N=373)	27	23	85	12
More than 10 years				
1965 (N=781)	19	33	65	20
1968 (N=368)	18	24	73	17

Although we cannot present the full data here, it should be emphasized that even though chronically ill patients were not as isolated from therapeutic programs in 1968 as they were in 1965 (Table 10-6), treatment patterns for those hospitalized more than five years still varied significantly among the four psychiatric units. For example, the proportions of such chronic patients receiving verbal therapy ranged from a high of 56 percent on the May unit to 45 percent on the Austin unit to 15 percent on the H-Complex to a low of 4 percent on the Dorchester unit.

The findings from the 1965 and 1968 treatment surveys can best be analyzed in relation to the organizational principle which asserts that the relevance and efficiency of an organization's throughput procedures determine its ability to convert environmental inputs into appropriate outputs. What do the data assembled from repeated treatment surveys at Boston State Hospital indicate about the relevance and efficiency of this organization's clinical technologies? Did the institution's inpatient-care subsystems, restructured via unitization, maximize the use of therapeutic rather than custodial technologies?

It is clear from our findings that change had indeed occurred in the anticipated direction, and that the hospital was emphasizing patient-centered treatment strategies. This is most strikingly evident in the staff's increased administration of drugs, with the result of reducing the percent of patients receiving no specific care from 37 percent in 1963 to 13 percent in 1968. Although data on hospitalwide treatment patterns in large psychiatric institutions will remain sparse until computerized studies such as that by Evenson et al. (1973) become more routinized, we believe that the extensive treatment program evident at Boston State Hospital compared quite favorably with that of similar institutions. Our findings outline the clinical technologies utilized by a changing mental hospital as it strived to react more effectively to community demands for changed outputs. The findings thus constitute a possible frame of reference for evolving judicial determinations regarding an institution's "adequacy of treatment."

In view of our conclusion that the increased administration of drugs, particularly to longterm and elderly patients, was the single most important factor in reducing the proportion of the hospital population receiving no specific therapy, it is meaningful to consider the implications of this technological emphasis. There had been wide acceptance among many Boston State Hospital staff of the clinical premise that inpatients, particularly chronic ones, have minimal interpersonal skills and inner capacities for coping with life's daily tasks; intensive verbal and activity therapies, therefore, were viewed as fundamental in helping psychotic individuals readjust to community living. Within this clinical perspective, the high level of drug therapy supported by the superintendent and social psychiatrically oriented staff was decried as being directed primarily toward patient management and symptom control. Yet, an increasing number of studies demonstrate the relative efficacy of drugs alone, or drugs plus psychotherapy, in the treatment of acute schizophrenics (May, 1968) as well as chronic ones (Grinspoon, Ewalt, & Shader, 1968). Although Feinsilver & Gunderson (1972) legitimately caution that these specific findings about drug effectiveness must still be restricted within one- and two-year time-limits of the drug's administration to patients, there can be little doubt that increasingly refined studies, such as that designed by Overall & Henry (1973), are impacting upon clinical practice. By contrast, the methodological morasses and ambiguities within which psychotherapy outcome studies remain enmeshed suggest that this technology's use with psychotic inpatients increasingly will be viewed as educationally valuable to the staff rather than clinically valuable to patients.

Can the changing purpose and utilization of psychotherapeutic interventions already be inferred from our data? At Boston State Hospital, which had been noted for its psychotherapy training program, our treatment surveys found that despite an improved patient-staff ratio the proportion of inpatients receiving verbal therapies had achieved a plateau, or decreased in absolute numbers, by 1968. Was this finding simply an artifact of the method used to define a patient's participation in verbal therapy, or did it indeed reflect the hospital's changing clinical practice?

Our operational definition of treatment—that the staff member has "a definite and continuing commitment for further work" with the patient—may have influenced our finding to some extent. This could particularly be the case in regard to the data indicating that far fewer patients participated in group psychotherapy in 1968 than in 1965. (Psychiatric residents reported only 23 patients in such groups at the latter point in time in contrast to the 174 patients included by them earlier.) Our operational definition of verbal treatment did not include within its scope the increased number of ward therapy programs initiated after the hospital's unitization in 1966. At least some of the patients who would have been counted in the 1965 survey as participating in more traditional and easily defined group therapy, in 1968 were being treated in more flexible, less easily measured ward programs.

It would be naïve, however, to conclude that the specific operational definitions utilized for research purposes alone produced the treatment plateau evident in the data about Boston State Hospital's 1968 verbal therapy activities. The role and nature of this clinical technology in the organization's total treatment effort was indeed being profoundly altered. No longer was it being provided in a standardized, clearcut manner, and less staff effort was being expended for this hitherto prestigious treatment of choice. For example, whereas 68 percent of the patients receiving individual psychotherapy in 1965 took part in two or more sessions a week, by 1968 only 32 percent of the individual psychotherapy patients received it that often. The declining, if not minimal, utilization of the psychotherapies in treating mental hospital patients has also been reported in such studies as that by Evenson et al. (1973). They found that more than half of the average 1.14 hours of individual therapy received by Missouri State Hospital patients was actually of the behavior-shaping type. Thus, we are led to suggest that the little psychotherapy being provided in mental hospitals increasingly is intended for the valuable purpose of staff education rather than direct patient benefit.

The third major clinical technology studied by the treatment surveys is the several activity therapies provided within psychiatric institutions. Considerable effort has been generated by mental hospitals during recent years to establish and expand a variety of rehabilitation services so that all patients would engage in treatment-oriented activities rather than simply lingering on custodial, antitherapeutic wards. The 1965 Boston State Hospital treatment survey found that 605 patients—32 percent of the total inpatient population—participated in one or more activity therapies. By 1968 the number of patients in these clinical services had dropped to 276, or 22 percent of the total population; a proportion towards the lower end of the involvement range reported by Linn (1970) in his nationwide study of patient participation in activities therapies at a sample of state mental hospitals.

In seeking the reason for the reduction at Boston State Hospital, we suggest that the key was the nature of the 1968 inpatient population. In general it was composed of less chronically ill and somewhat younger patients. Many of the better-functioning chronic patients had been discharged, and consequently the activity therapies in 1968 were involving only a limited hard core of regressed patients with whom staff had not even considered working earlier. Such patients need much more personal attention from rehabilitation counselors and occupational therapists because both their work and social skills have deteriorated. Thus, the activities therapies were no longer used extensively on all psychiatric services, but were more intensively concentrated on a small number of severely regressed patients.

In conclusion, we had asserted in our earlier description of an open systems approach to the study of organizational change (Chapter 4) that the throughput structures and processes utilized by a mental hospital are a key index of its ability to assume community mental health functions. This section's review of the changing clinical technologies employed at Boston State Hospital during the 1960s revealed that the community mental health goal of treatment for all rather than selected inpatients was being approached, primarily through the expanded administration of drugs. Although this changing technological emphasis has been decried by some analytically oriented psychotherapists, it is part of a larger clinical transition whereby the long-prestigious verbal therapies increasingly are being respected for their great value in training staff rather than for any intrinsic therapeutic benefit to psychotic inpatients. Such a modification of psychiatric throughput processes, thus, begins to correct what Polak (1971) has described as the irrelevance of hospital treatment focused upon the patient's intrapsychic concerns, when interventions directed, for example, at social system variables could be more beneficial to improving his coping ability and adjustment.

Finally, it is evident from even a superficial analysis of program developments throughout the country that within the next several years the current focus of concern will shift from simply insuring that therapeutic efforts replace custodial ones, to emphasizing quality control and program monitoring over the efforts directed at patients. Some of the complexities inherent in this process have been reviewed by Zusman (1972) and procedures are suggested by him for overcoming foreseeable problems. We can easily predict that despite the mental health professional's relative lack of experience in meeting the rigors imposed by sophisticated quality control, legislative and judicial pressures inevitably will require that psychiatric practices be subjected to the same scrutiny and critical review imposed upon other medical and human services specialties.

THE MENTAL HOSPITAL'S OUTPUTS

The survival and growth of a human services organization functioning as a people-belief-resource (PBR) system is very much related to its capacity for producing environmentally-desired outputs. The mental hospital, although such a PBR system, has been less constrained than most human services organizations to meet the demands of a market economy. It generally has succeeded in obtaining resources, albeit at a low level, despite societal dissatisfaction with its products, and has managed to survive under circumstances which normally lead to organizational dissolution. Longstanding societal ambivalence about the nature of the mental hospital's outputs obviously has fostered this state of affairs, but increasing emphasis by citizens upon community mental health principles slowly is altering this tradition. Mental hospitals are now being held accountable to generate acceptable products within an evolving framework of implicit and explicit criteria. Dissatisfaction with hospital outputs has even led California to plan the statewide closing of its public institutions by 1982 (Psychiatric News, 1973). Thus, our analysis of a changing mental hospital within the framework of open systems concepts must consider organizational outputs, as well as the inputs and throughput processes discussed earlier in this chapter. This additional analytic perspective is both theoretically meaningful and pragmatically useful for assessing institutional capacities to function as a community mental health center.

The study of organizational outputs has long been the cornerstone of program evaluation conducted within the goal attainment model. Despite the model's overemphasis upon the single organizational function as the measure of effectiveness (while disregarding input and throughput processes), outcome studies have gained wide professional and citizen acceptance. Sophisticated evaluations of psychiatric programs have been primarily conducted in relation to outcome alone, with little study of the associated input and throughput variables affecting systemic functioning. These analyses present easily understood formulations of cause and effect relationships and lend themselves fairly readily to statistical study.

The outputs of a community-oriented mental hospital may be defined as including discharged patients, trained personnel, change in health level among the community's population, research reports, patient maintenance programs, etc. Time constraints and limited personnel forced our study of Boston State Hospital to focus its outcome research upon the disposition of patient cohorts treated by the hospital at different points in time. This outcome analysis included two major studies: (1) the discharge pattern and characteristics of inpatients released from the hospital during the 1965–1968 period of major census reduction; and (2) a three-month follow-up of inpatients discharged to the local community.

Inpatient Discharge Patterns

Considerable attention has been attracted in recent years to the fact that throughout the country, mental hospital inpatient censuses have been dropping at accelerating rates. Our analysis of Boston State Hospital's residential population found the census decrease to be averaging 14 percent annually during the latter half of the 1960s (see Table 10-2). A lowered inpatient census can result from a reduced flow of admissions, a growing number of discharges, or both of these developments. Since Boston State Hospital's inpatient census decreased steadily during the 1960s despite a fluctuating number of admissions over this time-period (Table 10-2), the discharge pattern may be viewed as the key causal factor. What then are the variables associated with this discharge pattern, where did the patients go, and what personal and organizational characteristics were related to the patients' destinations?

The point prevalence surveys conducted in October 1965 and October 1968 of Boston State Hospital's inpatient population for the previously described treatment surveys had provided us with demographic data about all of the institution's residents at these two points in time. We thus could identify those individuals who had left the hospital between 1965 and 1968. Such an analysis revealed that only 598 members (32 percent) of the 1965 cohort of 1,880 inpatients were still institutionalized three years later. The remaining 1,282 inpatients (68 percent) had left the hospital during the interim. Since we lacked the resources to search the records of all 1,282 discharges, a 10 percent random sample was studied to determine outcome for the no-longer-hospitalized individuals. We specifically sought to determine whether the discharges had left the hospital for:

1. *Community living* arrangements such as their own home, a friend's home, day care or family care.
2. *Residential facilities* such as a nursing home, medical or psychiatric hospitals or the courts.
3. *Funeral homes* as the result of having died at Boston State Hospital.
4. *Other*, i.e., not yet officially discharged.

The case records of the dischargees revealed that less than one third of the group had left the hospital to resume independent or semi-independent community living arrangements (Table 10-7). A somewhat larger proportion (35 percent) had been discharged to other residential facilities (approximately three fourths of these to nursing homes), while the remaining third of the group had left the hospital via death. Given this differential discharge pattern for the sample studied, what patient variables were found to be determinants of outcome? The key characteristics affecting posthospital destination were found to be the individual's age and the length of time since his most recent admission to the institution, the same demographic variables which we had earlier shown to be basic determinants of the clinical technologies utilized in a patient's treatment (see Tables 10-5 and 10-6).

A highly significant difference was found in the discharge destinations of those individuals under age 60, and those 60 years and older (Table 10-8). The younger group returned primarily to community living arrangements or were transferred to other residential facilities. Very few died in the hospital. Among the elderly group, however, more than half left the hospital via death, another 41 percent were transferred to alternative residential facilities, and only 6 percent were able to resume

Table 10-7
Patient Destination Upon Discharge

Destination	*N*	%
Community living	35	29.2
Residential facility	42	35.0
Funeral home	40	33.3
Other	3	2.5
	120	100.0

Table 10-8
Age and Discharge Destination

Destination	*Age*			
	15-59		*60 +*	
	N	%	*N*	%
Community living	31	59.6	4	5.9
Residential facility	14	26.9	28	41.2
Funeral home	4	7.7	36	52.9
Other	3	5.8	0	0.0
	52	100.0	68	100.0

Chi square significant at .000 level

community living. A terminal outcome obviously is more actuarially likely among geriatric than nongeriatric inpatients, but it is important to stress that the elderly dying in the hospital were not simply cohorts of individuals with long histories of institutionalization, a common conception regarding those who pass away in this setting. Table 10-9 indicates a similar death rate among those hospitalized less than five years, and five years and more. The implication then is that mental hospitals, while overtly playing the role of treating the elderly in acute emotional distress, have in fact been used by society as terminal facilities for geriatric individuals with organic disorders. The question for the future is whether alternative community resources can be developed to care for such people, particularly as expanded insurance and medical benefits become available.

Our further finding that significantly more patients below age 60 than above age 60 returned to community living arrangements rather than alternative residential facililities (almost 90 percent of those aged 15–24 did so), may be viewed as reflecting the intrinsically greater capacity of the younger group to tolerate the daily

Table 10-9
Time Since Most Recent Admission and Discharge Destination

	Time			
Destination	*Less than five years*		*Five years and more*	
	N	%	*N*	%
Community living	28	47.4	7	11.5
Residential facility	9	15.3	33	54.1
Funeral home	21	35.6	19	31.1
Other	1	1.7	2	3.3
	59	100.0	61	100.0

Chi square significant at .001

stresses of open rather than sheltered environments. These data may also be analyzed, however, in relation to our previous finding that far greater hospital resources such as verbal and activity therapies were invested in treating younger than older inpatients (see Table 10-5). Were the observed age-related treatment patterns based upon differing initial diagnostic evaluations which then led to varied discharge outcomes (two thirds of those diagnosed neurotic or personality disorder returned to the community); or were the discharge outcomes independent of the hospital's technological interventions?

Although direct cause-effect linkages cannot be ascertained from the data in Table 10-10, chi-square analyses revealed that the specific treatment being received by a patient in 1965 was indeed significantly related to his posthospital destination. Half of the patients participating in verbal therapy returned to community living while only 20 percent of the 1965 patients not obtaining

Table 10-10
Type of Therapy and Discharge Destination

Type of Therapy	Destination									
	Community		*Residential Facility*		*Funeral Home*		*Other*		*Therapy Total*	
	(N=35)		(N=42)		(N=40)		(N=3)			
	N	%	N	%	N	%	N	%	N	%
None	3	12	9	36	13	42	0	0	25	100
Any Verbal	16	50	9	28	4	13	3	9	32	100
Any Activity	19	59	11	34	1	3	1	3	32	100
Any Somatic	28	34	29	35	25	30	3	1	85	100

such treatment displayed a similar outcome. Similarly, 60 percent of those participating in activity therapies subsequently returned to community living, while only 18 percent of those uninvolved in these therapies shared this outcome. Somatic therapy, which had previously been discussed in terms of its efficacy and growing utilization with psychotic individuals, was statistically unrelated to patients' post-hospital destination. The fact that various medications were administered to elderly patients for physical rather than psychiatric conditions, of course, confounds this particular analysis.

We had noted in earlier discussions of the mental hospital's efforts to reduce its backlog of chronic patients that various resources, particularly nursing homes, are being used as alternative caregivers for this population. The data in Table 10-9 and reports by Stotsky (1966, 1968) indicate that Boston State Hospital had developed extensive linkages to such facilities between 1965 and 1968. Over half of the patients discharged from the hospital after five years or more of institutionalization were placed in these residential alternatives. The return of longterm inpatients to community living arrangements was a relatively rare outcome during the period of this analysis despite the hospital's increased emphasis upon rehabilitation services and efforts to prepare these chronically ill individuals for new life patterns (Chien & Sharaf, 1971). Conversely, almost half of the patients hospitalized less than five years were found to have resumed community living patterns. This group, of course, included the younger individuals whose ability to function independently was still relatively intact.

In summary, our study of the modalities through which Boston State Hospital discharged two thirds of its 1965 inpatient cohort during the following three years, revealed that census reductions occurred through several outcome patterns. The return of patients to community living arrangements, the transfer of individuals to alternative residential facilities and the death of institutional residents comprised equally frequent routes through which inpatients departed the mental hospital. These routes were not randomly assigned or selected. They were clearly related to a patient's age and the length of time since his most recent admission to the hospital, the very same patient characteristics shown earlier as affecting the treatment pattern provided by staff. Younger, more recently hospitalized individuals had the best chance of resuming community living while older, longer-staying people more frequently were transferred to alternative residential facilities. Geriatric inpatients were at particularly high risk to die while residing in the institution regardless of length of time since admission.

Community Adjustment Patterns

The question of what happens to that group of individuals discharged from mental hospitals to community-based living arrangements has become a particularly gripping and vexing one during the past decade. It is being debated ever more vigorously as mental hospitals seek to reduce iatrogenic chronicity by retaining fewer and fewer individuals as inpatients. Proponents of deinstitutionalization emphasize the social breakdown syndrome of dependency and depersonalization fostered in people when they are isolated from community life for lengthy periods of time. Opponents of rapid deinstitutionalization vigorously cite the even more detrimental qualities inherent in the isolated living patterns being developed by discharged mental hospital patients (Lamb & Goertzel, 1971, 1972). Despite these often ideologic-like differences among professionals and citizens, the societal values of the 1970s, nevertheless, are swinging away from a longstanding reliance upon institutional care. It thus is crucial to determine what indeed occurs to those individuals discharged from mental hospitals into communities. Do the growing numbers of hospital "outputs" reflect increased organizational productivity and effectiveness, or are they simply statistical artifacts devoid of human significance? If the latter, what constructive measures can professionals and citizens take to avoid the predictable necessity for new minihospitals incorporating many of the same negative qualities found in larger phased-out institutions?

A Followup Study

The determination of a patient's adjustment subsequent to his discharge to a community living pattern involves complex conceptual issues, difficult methodological decisions, logistical deftness in adhering to data collection schedules, and sophisticated data analyses. May, Yale, & Dixon (1972) have reviewed these issues in some detail, and one can only marvel that rigorous followup studies such as those reported by Freeman & Simmons (1963) and Pasamanick, Scarpitti, & Dinitz (1967) are undertaken, persevered with and ultimately completed. Since our study of Boston State Hospital was an open systems analysis and focused upon a wide series of organizational variables in addition to the outcome of discharged patients, we were unable to conduct a followup survey with the detailed refinements appropriate to such research. Nevertheless, we did consider it essential to determine in even a sketchy manner the fate of persons discharged back to the community from unitized inpatient wards, and such a survey was performed in the spring of 1968.*

We described in Chapter 6 the manner in which Boston State Hospital initially unitized its inpatient services in 1966, and reported input, throughput and output data relevant to a cohort of individuals from the Dorchester sector of the hospital's catchment area. The followup study to be described here concentrated on the 75 persons admitted from this geographic sector as inpatients during March, April and May 1967, and who were subsequently discharged to community residential living arrangements. One-hour-long interview schedules were designed for the purposes of ascertaining 13 months after inpatient care was initiated, how patients and their significant others, i.e., relatives, perceived the hospitalization and discharge processes, the patients' functioning after return to community living and their utilization of community resources. Following a procedure whereby an experienced social worker initially contacted the significant other and then the patient, we succeeded in obtaining interview information about 42 (56 percent) of the eligible 75 patients (Table 10-11).

In any followup study, distinctions obviously exist between those patients who do and do not cooperate with the researcher. In this case, interviews were more likely to occur when the patient was female, Caucasian, over 40, not hospitalized prior to this episode, self- or family-referred to the hospital, had a longer stay, and had received aftercare. Even among the 42 cooperative cases, however, in only 16 instances was it possible to interview both the patient and the relevant significant other; for the other 26 cases interviews could be completed with

*The skill and diligence of Mrs. Joanne Marks in directing this effort is gratefully acknowledged.

Table 10-11
Followup Interviews on Patients (N = 75) Discharged to the Community

	N	%
Interviewed		
Patient Only	6	8
Significant Other Only	20	27
Patient and Significant Other	16	21
Total	42	56
Not Interviewed		
Not Located	17	23
Rejected Interview	16	21
Total	33	44

only the patient *or* a significant other. Almost all of the followup interviews with patients and the significant others were held in their homes; 16 percent were held at the interviewee's request in the researchers' offices or at Boston State Hospital.

Although the followup study's primary focus was upon a patient's adjustment to community-living posthospitalization, we deemed this outcome to be at least partially related to the patient's and significant other's perception of and attitude about the circumstances leading to the focal admission to Boston State Hospital. We determined through our interviews that, not surprisingly, patients and significant others judged these events from differing cognitive and affective perspectives. More of the patients than significant others considered hospitalization preventable; more significant others than patients judged the admission decision to be a correct one and felt relieved when it occurred. Thus, the strain experienced by patients and their families in living together also permeated the admission process and constituted but one more controversial issue requiring future clarification.

The psychiatrist's decision to admit an individual to inpatient care at a mental hospital may be based upon a variety of factors; highly salient among them is the need to provide the patient and his family with a respite from each other. Thus, the optimal length of hospitalization may be perceived differently by each party, depending upon his needs and restitutive capacities. However, psychiatric problems, treatment procedures and prognoses remain ambiguous, if not mystical, to many people; upon admission 50 percent of the patients and 31 percent of the relatives had no idea how long inpatient care would be required. The remainder anticipated that one month or less would suffice.

Length of hospital stay is generally thought to be determined by a patient's abilities and capacities (Altman et al., 1972), but it may also be based upon differing staff judgments about the consequences of discharge (Lorei, 1970) and degree of staff willingness to take risks in releasing marginally adaptive patients (Blackburn, 1971). The median length of stay for the cohort studied at Boston State Hospital was found to be 16.5 days, a duration deemed adequate by 68 percent of the patient-respondents and 53 percent of their significant others. On the other hand, 30 percent of the interviewed relatives judged their patients to have been discharged too soon, although only 14 percent of the patients expressed such a reaction. Virtually no patients or significant others considered the length of hospitalization excessive. Our followup interviews thus revealed that a majority of the patients and their families accepted the hospital's discharge timing as appropriate, while almost one third of the relatives deemed this action as premature. Since respite from a troublesome individual often is a basic motivation for the family's decision to seek his hospitalization, 30 percent of the families in the Boston State Hospital study may be viewed as expressing a lack of readiness for their relatives' return. This "acceptance-rejection" level is considerably better than that reported by Pokorny & Bentinck (1969) who found that only 20 percent of their patient sample were expected to return home by their relatives and that only 37 percent would have been welcomed if they did come home.

Another determinant of community adjustment by a discharged patient is whether he and his family perceive the inpatient treatment to have been a positive or negative experience; the former generates a constructive sense of growth and anticipation, while the latter fuels a sense of indignity and entrapment as the patient and his family resume the daily travails of living together. As in Kotin & Schur's (1969) similar study of the attitudes of discharged Boston State Hospital patients toward their inpatient experiences, we found that in 64 percent of the 42 cases studied, satisfaction was expressed by the patient and/or relative with the care received while the person was hospitalized; dissatisfaction was found in 31 percent of the cases, and 5 percent were undecided. The most frequent suggestion made to our interviewers was the need for greater staff involvement with patients and their families. Despite these reservations about the nature or quality of the hospital experience, we nevertheless found that in 86 percent of the 42 followed-up cases, the patient was thought by himself and/or his significant other to be improved as a result of inpatient care. In 7 percent of the cases the patient was considered unchanged, and in 7 percent he was deemed worse.

The followup interview data, thus, suggest that ambivalent reactions lingered among many significant others about the wisdom of the hospital's decision to discharge their relatives despite the preponderant judgment by relatives and patients that improvement had occurred in the patients' conditions. In view of the fact that many studies—e.g., Freeman & Simmons (1963)—have repeatedly demonstrated that family tolerance of bizarre behavior is a key factor in the posthospital outcome of discharged patients, we then turned to a review of the hospital's aftercare planning for these individuals. When the followed-up patients were asked what postdischarge treatment had been envisioned at the time of release, 91 percent stated that hospital staff had recommended aftercare patterns of drugs alone, verbal therapy alone or drugs plus verbal therapy. Only 9 percent of the patients couldn't recall a specific postdischarge treatment plan. Significantly, it was equally rare for the patients' families to be included in the planned community-based aftercare efforts.

Having reviewed patients' and significant others' perceptions of the hospitalization and discharge processes, we now will describe the adjustments experienced by these groups upon the patients' resumption of community activities. In terms of living patterns, we found at the time of followup interviews that two thirds of the patients had maintained the same residential arrangement as that engaged in prior to hospitalization. Thus, the majority had returned to settings shared with relatives; only a few were living alone. When patients were asked about their relationships with household members 13 months subsequent to the focal hospitalization, 52 percent judged the situation as improved, 28 percent perceived no change and 20 percent viewed it as worse. This last group included three individuals who were no longer living with spouses and whose marital status had changed to that of separated or divorced. Thus, the cohort selected for this followup study showed little deterioration in community living arrangements as the consequence of hospitalization, and more than half of it reported improved relationships with fellow household members, two key variables in assessing the quality of community adjustment by discharged patients.

A third variable widely deemed relevant to such an analysis is work status, i.e. whether the patient engages in employment after hospital discharge. Lorei (1970) had found that 81 percent of 1,254 Veterans Administration staff considered it at least moderately important that "the patient spend his time working or doing something useful after release." Lorei & Gurel (1973) have also reported, however, that extent of work in the preceding five years is the most useful prediction of posthospital employment so that it is difficult to anticipate significant improvement on this variable by patients who previously were unemployed. Table 10-12 indicates that when interviewed, 35 percent of the Boston State Hospital followup cohort was working while 62 percent was not employed. However, more than half of the latter group consisted of women who had not held jobs prior to hospitalization either. Thus, among the Boston State Hospital group, work status remained unchanged for two thirds of the cohort.

In addition to its psychological impact, hospitalization obviously also affects an individual's ability to maintain financial self-support. Did the inpatient experience modify our cohort's support sources when studied at the time of followup? Table 10-13 reveals that support sources for 55 percent of the group had remained unchanged, 10 percent were more independent financially, and 33 percent were more financially dependent subsequent to hospitalization. Among this last subgroup were a substantial number of individuals who now found themselves forced to rely upon various types of public funds even though this was not the case prior to the Boston State Hospital admission.

Table 10-12
Patient Work Status

Status	*Preadmission*				*Upon Followup*			
	Male	*Female*	*Total*	*%*	*Male*	*Female*	*Total*	*%*
Working	9	10	19	47.5	7	7	14	35.0
Not working	4	17	21	52.5	1	16	17	42.5
Hospitalized	0	0	0	0	4	4	8	20.0
Unknown	0	0	0	0	1	0	1	2.5
	13	27	40	100.0	13	27	40	100.0

Table 10-13
Patient Fiscal Support Sources

	Preadmission		*Upon Followup*	
Source	*No.*	%	*No.*	%
Wages only	12	30.0	9	22.5
Family only	13	32.5	9	22.5
Wages and family	5	12.5	4	10.0
Public funds only	5	12.5	14	35.0
Family and public funds	2	5.0	1	2.5
Wages and public funds	2	5.0	2	5.0
Unknown	1	2.5	1	2.5
Total	40	100.0	40	100.0

In view of our cohort's marginal work status, substantial dependence upon public fiscal supports and history of previous hospitalization (64 percent had experienced earlier inpatient care), the group obviously was at high risk to encounter future crises while adjusting to the rigors of community life. What psychosocial supports did they utilize, then, in the face of this possibility and how was this pattern related to the hospital's earlier aftercare planning? We found that 74 percent of the cohort had turned to an average of 2.4 community caregivers for assistance; medical resources were primary in this group but welfare help was also frequently sought. Although Boston State Hospital staff had planned continued contact with 91 percent of those discharged to the community, our interviews revealed that only half of these patients maintained a treatment relationship, usually in the form of visits to the drug aftercare clinic. The most common basis for reestablishing contact with hospital staff was found to be the patient's or significant other's concern about the need for possible inpatient readmission. Thus, we found that the studied cohort members actively reached out for primarily medical-type supports as they sought to stabilize their community adjustment, making relatively little use of the broader human services network potentially capable of assisting in this process. Whether the patient and his family, and/or the hospital's staff, were familiar with these additional resources, could not be determined.

Although replete with controversial conceptual and methodological implications such as those detailed by Morton et al. (1970), the decision to rehospitalize a psychiatric patient nevertheless remains a meaningful criterion of postdischarge adjustment by such individuals. Readmission also is a relevant index of the efficacy with which a community's aftercare network is or is not meeting the needs of the increased number of individuals being released from mental hospitals. Our followup study revealed that 53 percent of the 42 patients discharged from Boston State Hospital to community residential arrangements required further inpatient care within 13 months of the focal hospitalization; a majority of the readmissions occurred within three months of discharge. Unfortunately, this pattern is not dissimilar to that reported in many other studies, e.g., most recently by Hogarty et al. (1973), and it reflects the continuing turmoil being experienced by patients and their significant others as they anxiously grope for mechanisms to reestablish viable interpersonal relationships.

Finally, this brief but nevertheless revealing analysis of the community adjustment patterns displayed by a discharged cohort of Boston State Hospital patients sheds some light on the previously posed question about the meaning of increased hospital outputs. Our followup interview data indicate that postdischarge adjustment remains an anxiety-fraught experience for many of those studied; a not unexpected development in view of the fact that the focal hospitalization, the duration of inpatient care and even the nature of the treatment process are perceived somewhat differently by the patient and his significant other. Even though posthospital adjustment was abetted for many of our cohort members by a return to familiar residential settings shared with relatives, other traumas of family and community life prevailed in many instances. More than half of the cohort was rehospitalized within 13 months of the focal admission. Perhaps typical of the constricted lifestyle developed by these individuals is our finding that they sought aftercare support primarily within a familiar medical network. Although drugs and other medical services obviously are vital, these individuals' failure to seek out or to be referred to their community's relatively rich human services network for such assistance as social and recreational programs at least partially explains the marginal outcomes evident in our data.

SUMMARY

The earlier chapters of this open systems study of the changing mental hospital had reviewed the ideologic, administrative and resource utilization patterns employed by Boston State Hospital as it pursued community mental health goals. Our open systems analytic framework was specifically concerned with determining whether modified organizational practices affected patient care services, and this chapter has considered input, throughput and output measures relevant to the patients treated at this institution during the latter half of the 1960s. The information assembled through a variety of data collection procedures revealed that "people-processing" activities did indeed change during the time of our study.

In keeping with the hospital's intent to expand nonresidential treatment programs and to be perceived as more accessible to its community, increasing numbers of individuals were accepted for care by outpatient subsystems and fewer were admitted to inpatient units. Specific input patterns continued to vary with a person's age, race and marital status, but the hospital clearly was moving beyond the delimited, inpatient-focused concerns of its earlier history.

Our analysis of the treatment services provided inpatients demonstrated a clear increase in the number of individuals for whom a specific therapy was being provided. Furthermore, the assigned therapy was clearly related to the inpatient's age and length of time since most recent admission. While drugs grew in significance within the hospital's treatment activities and by 1968 were administered to 80 percent of the total inpatient body, individual and group psychotherapy were restricted to the 30 percent of inpatients in the lower age-categories who had been only recently hospitalized. Boston State Hospital's shifting "throughput" processes were also analyzed in terms of how effectively limited resources were deployed on an organizationwide basis so as to insure equal treatment opportunities for all rather than selected patients.

When the hospital's outputs were reviewed, we found that two thirds of the 1965 inpatient cohort had left the institution by 1968. Return to community living arrangements, transfer to alternative residential facilities and death in the institution were the virtually equally frequent routes through which inpatients departed the hospital. Once again, the variables of age and length of time since most recent admission were key determinants of specific release pattern. A followup study of the individuals discharged to community settings revealed that their adjustment during the subsequent months was an anxiety-fraught experience; more than half of this selected group was rehospitalized at least once within 13 months of the focal admission. The restricted range of aftercare and community services utilized by those studied is at least one indication of the difficulty experienced by such individuals as they seek to readjust to noninstitutional environments.

Section III

Human Services and Mental Hospitals

11. Human Services Systems: Does the Mental Hospital Have a Role?

Ten years have gone by since community mental health planning activities were initiated throughout the country. The past decade has been marked by intensive and purposeful, sometimes even frenzied, efforts to remodel our caregiving programs so that this period likely will be described by future historians as at once exhilarating, rewarding, frustrating and depressing for the professionals, citizens and clients associated with community mental health services. The positive memories will harken to the commitment which society made to those persons whom it had traditionally extruded, to the undaunted spirit with which recalcitrant problems were resolved and to the expanded network of community mental health facilities developed under the leadership of dynamic federal, state and local sponsors. However, negative recollections will also abound. Instead of President Kennedy's pioneering vision of a "bold new approach" to the care of the mentally ill, historians will recall the specter of anachronistically oriented administrators and clinicians adhering to the image of clients as passive and dependent persons rather than as resourceful and striving human beings, failing to alter hidebound practices and inappropriately vying for scarce resources.

It is within this framework of pride over significant accomplishments and dismay at lingering failures that we now complete this book by considering emerging human services program efforts for better meeting people's needs during the 1970s. Just as we started our work with an assessment of the factors specifically affecting the mental hospital's capacity to function productively during the community mental health era of the 1960s, so will we conclude this analysis by emphasizing the mental hospital's assets and liabilities during the emerging era of human services. Our assertions about such organizations are strongly colored, of course, by the preceding review of Boston State Hospital's changing functions and structures as it sought to achieve contemporary qualities. Our views are also predicated, though, upon events and developments throughout the country and, thus, are considered to have a broader and more valid basis.

The Concept of Human Services

There can be little doubt in the minds of even ardent skeptics that the manner in which mental health services are provided in the early 1970s differs significantly from the patterns of even a decade ago. Changes are evident in the conceptual rationales guiding program development as well as in the organizational arrangements through which services are offered to the public. The psychoanalytic precepts which guided the clinician's definition of problems and his assessment of treatment alternatives continue to be well-regarded, but no longer serve as the fundamental cornerstone upon which a mental health program is built. Social psychiatric concepts which recognize environmental influences as well as the principles of learning theory have become equally relevant for structuring clinical services and guiding personnel utilization. Outpatient community care rather than inpatient hospitalization is now the treatment of choice for acutely as well as chronically disturbed individuals. Furthermore, clinicians have come to accept the fact that they alone cannot resolve all behavioral problems and that the participation of other community caregivers, with varying degrees of sophistication, is essential to their mission. One result of this shift is that the provision of indirect services such as consultation is now a legitimate function of mental health agencies, and many professionals quite comfortably fill this role. As a result of the clinician's increased community orientation, local citizens have gained increased opportunities to help determine program priorities, and we are coming to respect the value of this previously unfamiliar input as well.

Although we recognize that the pace of these developments varies in different parts of the country, it nevertheless is clear that their general thrust is directed towards recognizing that a designated client's problems often are as much rooted in his community's tumultuous social structure and fragmented caregiving system as in his personal psyche. Human distress can be as profound when it results from unstable economic conditions and unresponsive social services as is the anxiety stemming from neurotic concerns and unresolved developmental crises. Inevitably, then, our contributions as mental health practitioners will always be severely limited if they do not fit into a broader context.

It is the definition of this broader context which is undergoing fundamental change. In the past decade our perspective and activities have expanded from the single purpose clinic or hospital to the more encompassing five essential services of community mental health programs. During the 1970s we will be challenged to evolve our scope even further by designing caregiving systems which provide clients with comprehensive and coordinated assistance of a nonpsychiatric as well as psychiatric nature. Human services systems will be concerned programmatically with health care, vocational training, rehabilitation, education, etc. From an administrative perspective, March (1968) and Demone (1974) have described these new human services systems as incorporating the following features: comprehensiveness, decentralized facilities located in areas of high population density, and integrated program administration which permits continuity of care from one service element to the next with a minimum of wasted time and duplication.

In examining the growth of human services programs, it is important to recognize the relationship between change and concepts. Often it is the case that real-world practices precede conceptual efforts to rationalize their validity, but it also is true that modified beliefs serve as an important precursor to action. Baker (in press) has suggested that the community mental health beliefs described in Chapters 3 and 7 as the prevailing ideology of the 1960s may well be supplanted by a human services ideology incorporating several new major attitude dimensions. Although the human services ideological structure is still emerging, the following five themes already characterize this belief system: systemic integration of services, comprehensiveness and accessibility, a problems-in-living definition of client troubles, helping activities containing generic qualities, and provider accountability to clients. The human services orientation is not viewed as incompatible with community mental health concepts; rather, it is an extension of these ideas through evolutionary processes. We would expect that just as those subscribing to sociotherapeutic beliefs could comfortably adapt to community mental health beliefs (Rabkin, 1972), so could these individuals also support a human services ideology even though each of these successive belief-systems is based upon ever-broader parameters of meaningful professional practice.

Just as we identified in earlier sections of this book

the relationship between community mental health ideology and clinical practices, so it is possible now to link human services concepts to local caregiving activities. For example, the increasing tendency to designate a community's variety of health and social welfare agencies as human services organizations reflects not only the desire to provide services more efficiently but also a growing societal as well as professional recognition of the common denominator inherent in the varied problems presented to us by clients. It also indicates an appreciation for the generic quality integral to the helping actions of professional and nonprofessional caregivers despite the multiple technologies utilized by them. The long-adhered-to distinctions between the problems germane to a psychiatric clinic and an alcoholism clinic, for example, or the traditional distinctions between the functions of different mental health professionals, have become increasingly artificial; many agencies have drastically revised their intake policies and clinical practices accordingly. Neighboring child guidance clinics and adult psychiatric clinics are being reorganized as family-oriented facilities, and agencies which previously excluded alcoholics, drug addicts and other special-problem cases now routinely accept individuals so troubled. Mental hospitals, which limited their services to psychiatrically defined problems, are undertaking such functions as aftercare programs to parolees from correctional institutions and residential care for runaway youths.

As mental health programs continue to extend their range of services, it will become all the more urgent that they forge systemic linkages with the other caregiving agencies needed to provide the complex array of resources, technologies and skills required for optimal client care. Defenders of the status quo need only follow a few clients through the present system in order to realize that it is poorly designed for resolving the multiple problems of those whom it purports to serve. The alcoholic client of a community mental health center may be offered outpatient psychotherapy, but little effort is made to arrange employment counseling or to involve his wife and children in the resolution of related familial problems. The parents of an emotionally disturbed child might well have to negotiate with the local psychiatric facility, the school system and the public welfare agency to insure that the youngster receives necessary educational and mental health services. Program coordination must also grapple with problems stemming from the fact that federal reimbursement for the identical service will vary according to whether it is provided by a health or social services agency.

Despite the erratic pace at which progress occurs towards resolving these problems, we are beginning to see concerted meaningful efforts to reorganize program components in such ways that they function more effectively than the currently fragmented caregiving network. At the heart of these efforts is an implicit, if not explicit, conceptual framework for helping people which recognizes that human services programs operate as a system of organizations whose participants are interdependent and must be appropriately linked (Baker & Schulberg, 1970; Boggs, 1972). Systems concepts, which have been used for the study of ecological relationships, increasingly are being applied to the design and operation of human services programs, and they are expected to be particularly relevant in defining the problems of management, of changing human services organizational goals, of interorganizational relations, and of organizational-environmental interaction. Chapters 2 and 9 reviewed the major contemporary systemic arrangements commonly known as the medical organizational and the human services networks, and their assets and limitations for achieving these purposes.

The application of systems concepts to the design and operation of human services programs represents an effort to optimize a rational, planned approach to the development of future caregiving arrangements. During the past decade planning has been sanctioned within given categorical fields such as health or social welfare, but with change occurring at an exponential rate the trend of the 1970s must be to broaden the planning base. Systems concepts are of singular value in expanding our grasp of a person's functioning and problems beyond the limited scope of a single categorical field so as to encompass a greater array of human services. They also highlight the fact that by shifting program emphases from one categorical sector to another, we upset delicate fiscal and personnel balances, which must then be reestablished.

The effectiveness of planning for human services, from an ecosystems perspective, is dependent upon the involvement and cooperation of the target community, the participation of established professional groups affected by potential program change and the sagacity of the planners themselves when faced with attractive alternatives in a turbulent environment. The temptation to run off simultaneously in all directions must be resisted. The planner of human services must understand that fundamental conflicts can be created if overly diverse philosophies, services and human inputs are incorporated within a single enterprise. He must determine whether administrative controls are to be vested in the professional or the community representatives, whether clinical-type services or social action are to be emphasized, and whether cooperative or conflictual strategies are to be utilized. Furthermore, the planner must distinguish between his short and longterm objectives since they may be antithetical—e.g., providing "new career" training to only some of the poor can be of immediate benefit to the trainees, but it may reduce poor people's support for the more fundamental and longrange changes needed to alter the poverty cycle. Choice selection is also becoming more complex as legislative actions compel human services to develop within the scope of broader urban undertakings, e.g., funds for corrections programs and preventive mental health activities are provided in the Safe Streets Act, and many social services are funded through Housing and Urban Development programs.

As the human services planner and administrator ponder these dilemmas and opportunities, their choices for program strategy can be guided by their definition of human problems and their causation.

1. The problem's definition. The characteristics and scope of human problems generally are defined by power groups and their societal agents rather than by affected populations. Although the definitions and optimal program strategies achieved from these differing vantage points may be congruent and lead to cooperative efforts, they may also be disparate and produce strife. For example, the drastic program changes undertaken by a leading New York family services agency stemmed from its board of directors' conclusion that individual casework could only minimally benefit the city's residents since the basic problem is really that of growing social ills afflicting whole neighborhoods rather than individuals alone. The board deemed its new view of the problem to be more congruent with that held by low-income and disadvantaged groups, and the problem redefinition permitted new program strategies such as court actions to be undertaken (Gottesfeld et al., 1973).

2. Theory of causation. Closely related to the problem's definition is the theory of its causation. Some theories are complex and multifactorial in nature and suggest the need for multiservice programs. Others are reductionistic and emphasize limited but intensive program efforts. For example, the poor achievement of minority groups in most public educational settings may be theorized as (a) stemming from insufficient preschool stimulation; (b) produced by the teacher's inability to understand children with cultural backgrounds and lifestyles different from her own; or (c) stemming from a combination of these and other factors. The first theory would emphasize compensatory preschool education for the children, the second would focus upon inservice training for school personnel, while the third would lead to a program strategy incorporating these two services as well as others—perhaps the busing of children to other school districts.

The training and selection of program personnel obviously are related to the underlying assumptions about the problem's definition, causation and distribution. In Chapter 2 we had considered the varying implications of the medical, public health and problems-in-living models for the provision of community mental health and human services. For example, problems with a singular cause affecting few people can feasibly be resolved by utilizing highly trained professionals to provide direct services and administer the total effort. When a problem is complex and affects large segments of the population, highly trained but inevitably limited numbers of professionals can only be used in selected ways, and difficult choices must be made.

The planning and administration of human services, thus, contain ever-broadening implications and possibilities. We must continue coping with any or all of these complexities: the lack of a definitive knowledge-base; alternatives whose feasibility is limited by statutory or fiscal constraints; selected, sometimes even entrenched, perspectives of providers and consumers; interorganizational competition for funds, staff and clients; and covert hostility towards client groups with selected racial and ethnic characteristics, or problems such as alcoholism and drug addiction. Additionally, the traditional distinctions between the roles and resources of a community's public, voluntary and private sectors have become increasingly blurred as decisions and dollars now flow across previously impermeable organizational and governmental boundaries at the local, state and national levels.

This overview of the contemporary health and social welfare scene suggests that a variety of conceptual, political, and administrative forces will affect human services programs, seeking to lead them in uncharted directions while simultaneously constraining them from moving too far from established patterns. Although these contradictory pressures create frustrating impasses and tenuous visions of the future, it still is possible to predict that during the coming decade human services programs and their affiliates will be required to redesign their operating practices, their manpower utilization patterns, their training procedures and their research foci. The details of these anticipated changes have been considered in depth by Schulberg (1972) and Schulberg, Baker, & Roen (1973), and they will be but briefly noted here.

Human services networks increasingly will focus on creating linkages between existing and planned organizations so as to facilitate client services, rather than seeking to incorporate all relevant services within a single agency. This approach recognizes that in most communities it will not be fiscally nor practically feasible for an individual facility to provide by itself all elements of a comprehensive program; in fact, some of the services may already be available elsewhere. The network approach is already evident in meeting the needs of such diverse populations as runaway youths and the elderly. After determining the basic needs of these groups and the essential services for meeting them, a consortium of agencies divides responsibilities according to their particular expertise. Many mental health centers have established comfortable and constructive roles within the framework of a human services network, particularly when their staffs are amenable to nonmedical contributions. The use of "interface teams," which include the staff of several agencies, to review specific cases has been particularly helpful in resolving outstanding problems and in fostering cooperative activities.

It is anticipated that categorical programs and facilities will become less common during the coming years and that comprehensive human services endeavors will expand. For this to occur, however, significant wide-ranging changes must be made within both organizations and individuals who traditionally have resisted even minimal departures from the tried and comfortable molds of the past. Ironically, the inertia of human services organizations has been reinforced on the one hand by bureaucratized administrative structures, professionalized personnel systems and relatively independent funding structures, and on the other hand by social values and priorities which change so rapidly and are so overwhelming that they are but tenuously considered.

The problem of manpower utilization is a particularly pressing one as human services grow since it is unlikely that increasing the number or professionals alone will modify the problems of maldistributed and improperly utilized personnel. Although it has become fashionable to recommend, as we did in Chapter 8, that instrumental roles based upon personal competency replace ascriptive roles related to professional degrees, the latter still continue to dominate the scene. New types of personnel at a variety of skill levels will be required, and distinctions among personnel in terms of salary and status can be related to such variables as the complexity of the client's problem, the required level of conceptual and technical skill, supply and demand, etc. Even more significantly, however, an overall training-service system must be designed within which individuals of varying ability can productively work towards common goals so that generalist and specialist skills are integrated within a cohesive framework.

IMPLICATIONS FOR THE MENTAL HOSPITAL

The mental hospital is one of the existing human services agencies which will be profoundly affected by the previously described trends. Even though it has survived many earlier attacks upon its existence, the mental hospital now is faced with an unparalleled crisis and challenge as it is subjected to fiscal and programmatic pressures. Many of the hospital's traditional functions such as custodial care and even acute treatment services are either anachronistic or better performed elsewhere. Diminishing inpatient censuses and the need to redeploy existing resources into high priority community-based services are leading many legislators and program administrators to question the current significant fiscal investment in psychiatric institutions. As new funding sources for expanding human services become increasingly difficult to obtain, the millions of dollars required to support mental hospitals become highly visible targets. Many planners and administrators are suggesting that the institutions be closed down, and a number of states already are implementing this policy despite the *Sturm und Drang* which it has provoked. Protests have emanated from those who argue, with considerable legitimacy, that some patients are being dumped in communities, that adequate alternative community facilities are lacking, that personnel rights are being abrogated, and that local economies are being disrupted. Nevertheless, the die has been cast, and the future role of mental hospitals already is the subject of intense scrutiny.

Chapter 2's review of the mental hospital's historic role in meeting the needs of disturbed individuals revealed that its position was not always an isolated or beleaguered one. In fact, for a period of time in the nineteenth century, the mental hospital movement embodied the same societal goals envisioned for community mental health programs in the 1960s. However, over the decades mental hospitals experienced many difficulties and failures in sustaining a therapeutic role, and their plight became increasingly worse during the first half of the twentieth century. Public and professional concern for the welfare of persons treated in these nontherapeutic institutions found expression in the late 1950s in the report of the Joint Commission on Mental Illness and Health. The resulting 1963 Community Mental Health Centers Act is deemed by many to have specifically intended that all mental hospitals be replaced by newly funded and operated local facilities. In fact, the recent Nader critique of the Act's accomplishments (Chu & Trotter, 1972) is very much predicated upon this interpretation of its original intent. However, it is clear that the federal goal of closing mental hospitals was neither subscribed to nor sympathized with in many parts of the country. The exigencies of financing, manpower needs and political pressures dictated that existing resources, including the mental hospital, be included in many of the local attempts to establish comprehensive community mental health programs. Federal funds for community mental health centers would be adequate to construct and staff only a small proportion of the needed facilities, and maximum utilization of existing local resources was crucial. It also became evident that metropolitan expansion and growing transportation networks had reduced the physical and psychological distance between many mental hospitals and their communities. The combination of these factors and others led many states to conclude by 1965 that the luxury of disregarding the mental hospital's potential as the core or major component of certain comprehensive programs could not be afforded. In many instances, therefore, mental hospitals were mandated to provide the five essential services to their own local areas as well as to provide additional services for which they were uniquely staffed and/or equipped.

We now must assess the results of a public policy designed to utilize the mental hospital as a contemporary, therapeutic facility. Such an evaluation of organizational relevance and effectiveness is difficult under the best of circumstances, as was noted in Chapter 4 and by Baker & Schulberg (1973), and it has been made even more complex by the fact that the assessment criteria now extend beyond the question of the mental hospital's functioning as a community mental health center and include variables pertinent to its potential as a human services resource. It is clear that the present parameters for defining a community mental health center's clients and services are in flux because of changing societal assumptions about client need, shifting funding patterns and swelling demands for service. Caregivers, consequently, are being pressured to modify the systemic concepts and organizational linkages within which they function and to assume broader programmatic obligations.

Given this evolving analytic framework for assessing the mental hospital's future as a viable human services resource, the resulting picture is at best a mixed one. There are many who contend that the existing psychiatric institutions remain as outmoded today as they were in the past. Others fervently profess that these facilities continue to warrant societal and legislative support. What are the facts and rationales behind these contradictory assertions and how will they influence future program developments? The remainder of this chapter will consider the mental hospital's viability as a contemporary human services agency and suggest directions to which it must turn if it is to survive through the 1970s.

Input Projections

Any forecast of the mental hospital's fate obviously must pay heed to the nature and volume of its inputs during the coming years. For which individuals will society seek care and treatment in such facilities, and with what frequency will such persons be admitted to these institutions? How are these epidemiologic projections affected by developments within a mental hospital and the broader human services network of which it is a component? Our intensive study of Boston State Hospital's transition to a community mental health center found that changing clinical programs within the institution were related to altered client input patterns from the geographic catchment area and to modified clientele selection priorities (Chapter 10). Do these findings from one urban community and its mental hospital reflect a unique situation in a large New England city, or can they be considered as suggestive of wider trends?

The literature reports that inputs to the mental hospital indeed are changing throughout the country, in rate and nature of clientele and in the services provided them. A review of national mental health program trends by Ozarin & Feldman (1971) found a drastic 33 percent reduction in state hospital populations between

1955 and 1970, as well as a shift in the focus of care from inpatient to outpatient service. In 1955, 71 percent of patient care episodes occurred in hospitals and 22 percent in outpatient clinics. In 1968, the figures were 43 percent for hospitals and 45 percent for clinics.

The decreased need to utilize the residential facilities of mental hospitals generally is associated with the advent of tranquilizers in the mid-1950s, but the growth of community mental health centers in the 1960s has lent further impetus to this trend. Stubblebine & Decker (1971) and Wolford et al. (1972) detail the manner in which state hospitalization rates were reduced in San Francisco and Pittsburgh, respectively, as expanding community mental health programs assumed greater responsibilities. In the former city involuntary patients were treated locally because the Superior Court and the mental health services were determined to substitute local care for mental hospital commitment. The result was the virtual disappearance of institutional commitments.

An example of how shifting definitions of human problems and their causative factors affect input projections to human services networks in general, and mental hospitals in particular, is the movement by many states to define alcoholism as a medical rather than criminal problem. This shifts the locus of responsibility to health and social welfare services away from correctional ones. Although the mental hospital may be initially required to provide added detoxification and rehabilitative services for an increased clientele, it is quite likely that as additional federal and state funds become available other community caregivers such as general hospitals and sheltered workshops will subsequently assume many of these responsibilities. Holder & Stratas's (1972) description of a systems approach to alcoholism programming indicates the alternatives in designing comprehensive alcoholism networks, which may or may not include the mental hospital's resources. Thus, although alcoholics already comprise approximately one third of mental hospital admissions and their number may temporarily rise even higher, it is likely that as community alternatives evolve over a period of years the number of alcoholics served by mental hospitals will dwindle.

While more and more planners project the diminished use, even the abandonment, of mental hospitals in treating a community's emotionally disturbed residents, other experts emphasize the continued need for these facilities in caring for the chronically ill. Few dispute that these individuals will always represent a sector of the community's psychiatric caseload. Whether their needs can be met through community mental health centers and other resources, or whether mental hospitals are needed, is a key ambiguity in forecasting future program trends. Reports such as those by Kraft et al. (1967) about the Fort Logan Community Mental Health Center, and Myerson (1972) about Worcester State Hospital, assert that chronic, unresponsive schizophrenics accumulate and constitute a substantial portion of a facility's treatment population despite efforts to avoid this "silting." All would agree that specialized input and treatment procedures are needed for these individuals, but there is less consensus as to whether these procedures are best organized and administered within the framework of mental hospitals.

Along with this significant uncertainty about our ability to dispense totally with mental hospital services in treating traditionally defined psychiatric clients, countertrends at some psychiatric institutions raise additional questions about the universality and inevitability of the declining volume of client inputs to mental hospitals. It is evident that given proper statutory and administrative sanctions, institutions located in urban centers and capable of establishing links to the local human services system can generate major changes in the clients for whom they accept responsibility. At a number of Massachusetts institutions such as Boston State and Worcester State Hospitals, the range of community-oriented services was expanded as the psychiatric custodial censuses dwindled. Consequently, previously ignored populations like drug addicts and runaway youth are now being admitted for care. If the expanding clientele and program trends of psychiatric institutions continue in such directions, mental hospitals will in point of fact be accepting the very inputs deemed characteristic of human services centers. Their clientele will include individuals with a variety of social and physical problems, and the category of individuals whom we now define as psychiatrically ill will be but one of those served by these emerging centers.

This expanded view of the mental hospital's potential future inputs clearly stems from the premise discussed earlier in this chapter—i.e., that there are sufficient common denominators in the personal needs of the psychiatrically disturbed, the parolee, the physically handicapped, the alcoholic, etc.—that they can receive a variety of general as well as unique services within a single comprehensive caregiving facility staffed by generalists. Conversely, if these client populations are viewed as having specific needs which can best, or only, be met in a categorical service center staffed by trained and experienced professionals, it is unlikely that they will be perceived as appropriate inputs for changing mental hospitals.

Program Options

This beclouded vision of a community's options and intentions for meeting diverse citizen needs produces differing forecasts of whether mental hospitals are to be incorporated within future human services networks. At the one extreme is the contention by many observers that most mental hospitals in urban as well as rural settings have failed to significantly modify their program philosophy and operating practices. These observers assert that although these institutions may have eliminated the worst characteristics of the snakepit era, they have undertaken very few of the programmatic changes essential to contemporary functioning. The 1971 decision of a federal court in the case of *Wyatt v. Stickney*, requiring Alabama's mental hospitals to upgrade services, reveals the desperate situation which still exists in at least some of our psychiatric institutions.

In a variety of instances, the mental hospital's failure to meet contemporary standards has resulted from a state's policy decision to expand community-based services and to phase out institutions. In other instances, the hospital's own personnel have lacked the leadership required to develop and administer progressive programs even when given the mandate to do so. An even more fundamental issue about the mental hospital's viability is that raised by Mendel (1968) and Polak & Jones (1973), who contend that existing mental hospitals by definition are antitherapeutic; by admitting troubled persons, they permit communities to avoid mobilizing the social and psychological support systems which these persons require. Many also question the assumption that deviant behavior can better be assessed and diagnosed in the hospital than in the person's natural environment. From this perspective it is clear that regardless of whether the hospitals' limited progress is societally determined or organizationally induced, many existing institutions are not meeting people's needs; that they should be phased out; and alternative provisions must be sought for the clientele whom they traditionally have served.

More optimistic prognoses of the mental hospital's future stem from the viewpoint that many of these facilities already are, or still are, capable of making constructive contributions to a community's need for the full spectrum of human services. Overviews by Ozarin & Levenson (1969) and Greenblatt (1971) point to several contemporary roles within the psychiatric institution's grasp, e.g., serving as the core of a health system or undertaking community mental health functions within a larger caregiving network. This book has focused upon the issues and strategies, successes and failures of Boston State Hospital as it evolved from its traditional role as an inpatient-oriented psychiatric institution to its now more broadly conceived role as a community mental health center. A similar approach to the hospital's future program structure, very much based upon the conceptual models described in Chapter 2, is offered by Fisher, Mehr, & Truckenbrud (1973). They suggest dividing the institution into three sectors: (1) a Medical-Freudian section for persons with physical disorders that clearly are causing behavioral reactions; (2) a Voluntary Human Services section for persons who cannot function in traditional community settings; and (3) an Involuntary Security section for people who do not seek admission but whose behavior violates the right of others.

A more circumscribed but, nevertheless, significant contribution to meeting a community's human services needs through mental hospital facilities is suggested by Bartz, Loy, & Cook (1971). They view psychiatric institutions as caring only for those special populations which cannot be accommodated within community mental health centers, e.g., alcoholics, acting-out adolescents, chronic no-family persons and those dangerous to others. Bartz et al. view existing mental hospitals as appropriate residential settings for these populations since their treatment requires total-control environments in which intensive behavioral training and change can occur.

Even these optimistic forecasts must be tempered, however, by the recognition that despite positive societal mandates and creative leadership efforts, many well-intentioned mental hospitals may be unable to overcome the legacies of deteriorating physical plants and staffing patterns inappropriate to contemporary programs. The first problem is poignantly exemplified at Boston State Hospital. Over the past decade, this organization has given top priority to improved patient care and treatment environments and has moved in the various program directions described earlier in this book despite the profoundly constraining influence of poor plant conditions. In February 1973, however, the superintendent was forced publicly to acknowledge that "Boston State Hospital is physically dying." Capital improvement funds were again sought from the state legislature after the Joint Commission on Hospital Accreditation rescinded the hospital's accreditation because its toilets and lighting were so bad. The superintendent warned that if these physical conditions were not quickly remedied, staff would be lost and programs and patient care surely would deteriorate despite the hard-won gains of the past decade.

An equally frustrating dilemma in insuring the mental hospital's program growth is that of establishing personnel patterns appropriate to contemporary purposes. An analysis of staff employed at the Massachusetts mental hospitals in 1973, for example, revealed that although staff-patient ratios generally exceeded the earlier goal of 1:1, the present problem is that of limited treatment personnel and excessive custodial and maintenance personnel. This situation is illustrated by the fact that more than four times as many employees were maintaining Massachusetts hospital buildings and grounds as there were psychiatrists, psychologists and social workers combined to treat the patients residing within them. Similarly, even in the face of the 1972 *Wyatt* v. *Stickney* court order to upgrade personnel patterns, the director of an Alabama mental hospital has acknowledged that "the volume of skills is not available and not likely to be available until Alabama establishes competitive pay grades and appropriates the necessary funds" (*Psychiatric News*, 1973b).

The mental hospital's program options for the 1970s, thus, include the choice of (1) abandoning the ghost of relevance and closing down; (2) assuming highly specialized functions which cannot be performed elsewhere; and (3) undertaking fullscale human services activities. We must reiterate, however, that even when new mandates are achieved and contemporary directions pursued, the constraints of antiquated physical facilities and inappropriate staffing patterns stand ready to thwart progress.

Planning for Mental Hospitals

A decision about the mental hospital's future, given the previously cited range of options, must include complex considerations such as community alternatives, client need, staff capability and fiscal support. Careful planning efforts obviously are warranted before action is undertaken. These analyses already have been called for in the Nader Report, which chose to emphasize that "planning should immediately be initiated for the long-range demise of state hospitals" (Chu & Trotter, 1972). Statewide planning efforts similar in scope and significance to the early 1960s projects described in Chapter 1 have recently been conducted in such states as Massachusetts (Schulberg, 1973) and California (*Psychiatric News*, 1973a), and it is meaningful to consider the approaches they have taken and the reactions they are meeting in seeking to implement program and facility modifications.

An organization's future role and viability can be assessed along a variety of dimensions. When the mental hospital's future is considered, planning can focus upon either (1) the hospital's clients or (2) its organizational capacities. The first approach scrutinizes the needs of those currently being served by public psychiatric institutions and determines whether better alternatives do or will exist elsewhere. This planning strategy relies heavily upon data of the types described earlier in this chapter regarding the community's projected input patterns, and it is particularly concerned with the use of public policy in altering utilization patterns of diverse human services facilities. It is entirely conceivable from this analytic perspective to recommend the phased closing of all mental hospitals as community-based alternatives to largescale institutions are established. The second planning approach primarily focuses upon organizational strengths and weaknesses, and places relatively less emphasis upon alternative options to the mental hospital. Although not intended as such, planning which focuses upon mental hospitals rather than the people they serve often leads to a preoccupation with organizational maintenance rather than optimal client benefits and improved systemic caregiving patterns.

The 1972–1973 Massachusetts effort to plan for the future of its public mental hospitals decided to focus initially upon the several populations then being served within these institutions. By determining their clinical needs and assessing the optimal public and voluntary service systems required to provide appropriate care, one could then judge whether the mental hospital had any longterm role. Planning, therefore, reviewed client characteristics, treatment technologies and facility requirements in treating the adult mentally ill, geriatrics, adult psychiatric offenders, children and youth, and addictions. This planning approach can be illustrated by a brief description of the issues raised and recommendations made about the first of these populations, and the implementation procedures which then would ensue.

Adult Mentally Ill

The adult mentally ill have long been the major population cared for in mental hospitals, and it is around their gross needs and abilities that most institutional programs were designed. This organizational emphasis usually had resulted in the construction of major inpatient psychiatric services, and it is only in the past decade or two that we have come to recognize the finer and subtler clinical needs of those persons who traditionally occupied these beds. Consequently, a planning approach to the needs of the adult mentally ill must consider the distinctions between those individuals requiring (1) acute intensive treatment, (2) longer-term community-based care and (3) continued institutional care.

Although the mental hospital has long been used for and occupied by all three of these groups, the current thinking of many professionals is that the first two groups of adults can better be treated in facilities other than the mental hospital and that the third group is rapidly diminishing in size. This position is based upon the rationale that community-based care is preferable to that in mental hospitals because it fosters the integration of emotionally disturbed individuals into the mainstream of normal life and diminishes disability and dependency. This position maintains that institutional settings tend to be depersonalizing and lacking in accountability regardless of how superior the leadership efforts may be. Therefore, communities must be encouraged to accept total responsibility for their mentally ill, and this will occur only if extrusion to distant mental hospitals is no longer possible. If we assume that (1) the clinical needs of acutely ill adults can be met through such community facilities as the general hospital and (2) longterm chronically hospitalized individuals can be placed in various community residences, it is indeed possible to project a caregiving network for the adult mentally ill which no longer utilizes the mental hospital.

There are many professionals and citizens, to be sure, who view such a program policy for the adult mentally ill as premature if not naïve. They contend that it still is not possible to maintain the chronically ill in communities and that to preclude the availability of mental hospital facilities is deleterious to the welfare of such individuals. This position is based upon evidence of continuing high readmission rates for those discharged from mental hospitals; a consistent unwillingness by many cities and towns to permit the establishment of community homes for the mentally ill in residential neighborhoods; and growing concern about neurological disorders stemming from prolonged use by chronic schizophrenics of neuroleptic drugs (Crane, 1973). Nevertheless, these cautionary tones have not impeded public policy recommendations opposing continued use of institutional facilities, and steps are being initiated in Massachusetts and other states to minimize and eliminate mental hospital services for the adult mentally ill.

Implementation Procedures

It already is evident that similar recommendations are or will be made about utilizing alternatives to the mental hospital for treatment of the other clinical populations now being served in these institutions. It, therefore, is necessary to consider the implementation issues and decisions which will confront program administrators undertaking transitions of this scope and complexity. We will first address the fiscal dilemma because of its central importance. The noninstitutional human services network will require significant expansion as it assumes previous mental hospital responsibilities and since fiscal austerities in 1973 preclude the expectation that additional funds will be forthcoming from state or federal governments to augment these community-based services, resources being spent for mental hospital support inevitably will have to be redeployed into alternative caregiving organizations if they are to flourish. The simplicity or complexity of fiscal redeployment will vary among states, depending upon local budget-setting procedures and degree of legislative control over allocations.

In states where community fiscal autonomy exists, Schulberg (1973) has suggested that as a possible first step public funds not be directly appropriated to mental hospitals but rather to designated citizen groups charged with the responsibility for purchasing those comprehensive services pertinent to the needs of local residents. Assuming that appropriately high standards can be imposed and maintained, the citizen group would have the prerogative of purchasing human services from whatever resource it deems most effective, thus placing client need before provider interests. If the customer has a choice in purchasing psychiatric and other services, the budget of a mental hospital would then have to be supported through the services which it sells in an open market to those mental health and nonmental health, public and private programs which choose to utilize its resources. If the mental hospital can offer an appropriate product and attracts customers, it will survive; if it cannot compete in an open economic market, then it should not be maintained. A strict purchase of service approach to human services programming admittedly produces problems, e.g., local human services administrators may decide to purchase clinical care solely upon the basis of cost rather than quality. This fiscal strategy could also jeopardize the minimal level of organizational stability needed to insure program continuity. Nevertheless, it represents an attractive initial alternative to our present budgetary mechanisms which often maintain programs out of traditional rather than functional concerns. This strategy thus deserves further consideration, particularly if it can be combined with a plan for adjustable base subsidies along the lines suggested by Boggs (1972).

Another key issue affecting the redesign of mental health and human services efforts is the need to help local citizens and program administrators accept responsibility for not only the clients whom they traditionally viewed as coming within their purview, e.g., neurotics and depressives, but also for those persons formerly perceived as falling within the mental hospital's jurisdiction, e.g., chronic schizophrenics and the aged. Furthermore, the individual needs and job security of mental hospital employees must be viewed with respect rather than disdain if labor's support is to be enlisted in the task of implementing contemporary caregiving systems. Although each of these policy and program issues is formidable and not easily resolved, the evidence is growing that a public and steadfast commitment to new service delivery mechanisms can achieve success in better meeting clients' needs. New programs can be established for those previously served by psychiatric institutions (e.g., Oberleder, 1973), and organizational problems associated with the closing of a mental hospital can be overcome (e.g., Stewart et al., 1968; Mosher & Gunderson, 1973). The human services administrator's willingness to battle societal and professional resistance to deinstitutionalization is, of course, a sine qua non in these efforts, and upon his fortitude rests the nature of future community programs for the mentally ill and emotionally disturbed.

SUMMARY

The conceptual and caregiving framework within which clients' problems are resolved has expanded in recent years to include nonpsychiatric as well as psychiatric concerns. New human services systems are developing with an emphasis upon comprehensiveness, decentralized facilities and integrated program administration insuring continuity of care. The implications for the mental hospital are profound and challenge its continued viability. It already is evident that given proper statutory and administrative sanctions, mental hospitals capable of establishing links to the local human services system can undergo major changes in clients and functions so that within a period of years they will be functioning as human services centers. Other mental hospitals which for societally determined or organizationally induced reasons are not functioning within a contemporary framework of systemically related human services should be phased out and closed. These decisions are complex ones dependent upon projected client utilization patterns, alternative community-based resources, options for fiscal redeployment and personnel prerogatives. Nevertheless, a commitment to providing clients with optimal services must remain the basic motivation for pursuing change, and the mental hospital's future should be resolved only within this framework.

References

Ackoff, R. Systems, organizations, and interdisciplinary research. *General Systems Yearbook*, 1960, **5**, 1–8.

Acock, A. & DeFleur, M. A configurational approach to contingent consistency in the attitude-behavior relationship. *Amer. Sociological Review*, 1972, **37**, 714–726.

Adorno, R., Frenkel-Brunswick, E., Levinson, D., & Sanford, R. *The authoritarian personality*. New York: Harper & Row, 1950.

Almond, R. & Kupfer, D. Psychiatric inpatient research. *J. Nerv. Ment. Dis.*, 1969, **149**, 398–407.

Altman, H., Angle, H., Brown, M., & Sletten, I. Prediction of length of hospital stay. *Comp. Psychiatry*, 1972, **13**, 471–480.

American Psychiatric Association. *Standards for psychiatric facilities*. Washington, D.C.: American Psychiatric Association, 1969.

Armor, D. & Klerman, G. Psychiatric treatment orientations and professional ideology. *J. Hlth. & Soc. Behavior*, 1968, **9**, 243–255.

Auerswald, E. Changing concepts and changing models of residential treatment. In G. Caplan, & S. Lebovici (Eds.), *Adolescence: Psychosocial perspectives*. New York: Basic Books, 1969. Pp. 343–357.

Ayllon, T. & Azrin, N. *The token economy: A motivational system for therapy and rehabilitation*. New York: Appleton-Century-Crofts, 1968.

Babow, I. & Johnson, A. Staff attitude profiles and response to an administrative innovation in a mental hospital. *Nursing Research*, 1968, **17**, 269–273.

Baker, F. An open-systems approach to the study of mental hospitals in transition. *Comm. Ment. Hlth. J.*, 1969, **5**, 403–412. (a)

Baker, F. Review of general systems concepts and their relevance for medical care. *Systematics*, 1969, **7**, 209–229. (b)

Baker, F. General systems theory, research, and medical care. In A. Sheldon, F. Baker, & C. McLaughlin (Eds.), *Systems and medical care.* Cambridge, Mass.: MIT Press, 1970. Pp. 1–26.

Baker, F. The changing hospital organizational system: A model for evaluation. In M. Rubin (Ed.), *Man in systems*. New York: Gordon & Breach Science Publishers, Inc., 1971. Pp. 323–337.

Baker, F. Planning and the environment of a community mental health center. *Psychiat. Quart.,* 1972, **46**, 95–108.

Baker. F. Organizations as open systems. In F. Baker (Ed.), *Organizational systems: General systems approaches to complex organizations.* Homewood, Illinois: Richard D. Irwin, 1973. Pp. 1–25.

Baker, F. The living human service organization: Applications of general systems theory and research. In H. Demone & D. Harshbarger (Eds.), *A handbook of human service organizations.* New York: Behavioral Publications, 1974. (a)

Baker, F. From community mental health to human service ideology. *Amer. J. Pub. Hlth.*, in press.

Baker, F., Broskowski, A., & Brandwein, R. Systems dilemmas of a health and welfare council. *Social Service Review*, 1973, **47**, 63–80.

Baker, F. & O'Brien, G. Intersystems relations and coordination of human service organizations. *Amer. J. Pub. Hlth.*, 1971, **61**, 130–137.

Baker, F., O'Brien, G., & Sheldon, A. Reference group orientations of occupational therapists at a changing mental hospital. *Amer. J. Occupational Therapy*, 1968, **22**, 197–202.

Baker, F. & Schulberg, H. The development of a community mental health ideology scale. *Comm. Ment. Hlth. J.*, 1967, **3**, 216–225.

Baker, F. & Schulberg, H. Community mental health ideology, dogmatism, and political-economic conservatism. *Comm. Ment. Hlth. J.*, 1969, **5**, 433–436.

Baker, F. & Schulberg, H. Community health caregiving systems: Integration of interorganizational networks. In A. Sheldon, F. Baker, & C. McLaughlin (Eds.), *Systems and medical care.* Cambridge, Mass.: MIT Press, 1970. Pp. 182–206.

Baker. F. & Schulberg, H. A system model for evaluating the changing mental hospital. In F. Baker (Ed.), *Organizational systems: General systems approaches to complex organizations*. Homewood, Illinois: Richard D. Irwin, 1973. Pp. 476–488.

Baker, F., Schulberg, H., & O'Brien, G. The changing mental hospital—Its perceived image and contact with the community. *Ment. Hyg.*, 1969, **53**, 237–244.

Baker, F., Schulberg, H., Yager, J., & O'Brien, G. Problems of a centralized department in a decentralized mental hospital. *Soc. Sci. & Med.*, 1970, **4**, 239–252.

Bartz, W., Loy, D., & Cook, W. Mental hospitals and the winds of change. *Ment. Hyg.*, 1971, **55**, 266–269.

Bay, A. Discussion of Dr. Smith's paper. *Mental Hospitals*, 1964, **15**, 74–75.

Becker, A., Wylan, L., & McCourt, W. Primary prevention—Whose responsibility? *Amer. J. Psychiat.*, 1971, **128**, 412–417.

Belknap, I. *Human problems of a state mental hospital.* New York: McGraw-Hill, 1956.

Bellak, L. *Community psychiatry and community mental health*. New York: Grune & Stratton, 1964.

Bennis, W., Berkowitz, N., Affinoto, M., & Malone, M. Reference groups and loyalties in the outpatient department. *Admin. Sci. Quart.*, 1958, **4**, 481–500.

Bertalanffy, L. von. The theory of open systems in physics and biology. *Science*, 1950, **111**, 23–28.

Bertalanffy, L. von. General systems theory. *General Systems Yearbook*, 1956, **1**, 1–10.

Blackburn, H. Factors affecting turnover rates in mental hospitals. *Hosp. Comm. Psychiat.*, 1971, **23**, 268–271.

Bockoven, J. Moral treatment in American psychiatry. *J. Nerv. Ment. Dis.*, 1956, **124**, 167–194.

Bockoven, J. The moral mandate of community psychiatry in America. *Psychiatric Opinion*, 1966, **3**, 32–39.

Boggs, E. The mad tea party: An ecological approach to changing human service systems. Paper presented at Institute on Hospital and Community Psychiatry, St. Louis, Mo., September 26, 1972.

Bolman, W. Community control of the community mental health center. *Amer. J. Psychiat.*, 1972, **129**, 173–186.

Bonn, E. & Kraft, A. Fort Logan Mental Health Center: Genesis and development. *J. Ft. Logan Mental Health Center*, 1963, **1**, 17–27.

Boyles, P. & Waldrop, G. Development of a community-oriented program in a large state hospital of limited resources. *Amer. J. Psychiat.*, 1967, **124**, 29–31 (Oct. Supp.).

Breeskin, J., Wolff, S., & Witzke, D. Community mental health ideology in the military. Presented at the 19th Annual Conference of Air Force Behavioral Scientists, January 1972.

Brill, H., Folson, J., St. Pierre, R., & Zubowicz, G. The

unit system of operation. *Mental Hospitals*, 1963, **14**, 117–118.

Brill, H. & Patton, R. Analysis of population reduction in New York State mental hospitals during the first four years of large-scale therapy with psychotropic drugs. *Amer. J. Psychiat.*, 1959, **116**, 495–508.

Burdock, E., Glass, L., Hardesty, A., & Beck, Y. A sample survey of mental hospital patients. *J. Clin. Psychol.*, 1961, **17**, 253–259.

Burling, T., Lentz, E., & Wilson, R. *The give and take in hospitals.* New York: Putnam, 1956.

Burris, D. (Ed.) *The right to treatment.* New York: Springer, 1969.

Caplan, G. *Principles of preventive psychiatry.* New York: Basic Books, 1964.

Caplan, G. & Caplan, R. Development of community psychiatry concepts in the United States. In A Freedman & H. Kaplan (Eds), *Comprehensive textbook of psychiatry.* Baltimore: Williams and Wilkins, 1966. Pp. 1499–1516.

Caplan, R. with Caplan, G. *Psychiatry and the community in nineteenth-century America.* New York: Basic Books, 1969.

Caudill, W. *The psychiatric hospital as a small society.* Cambridge, Mass.: Harvard University Press and Commonwealth Fund, 1958.

Chien, C. & Sharaf, M. Factors in the discharge of chronic patients. *Hosp. Comm. Psychiat.*, 1971, **22**, 236–238.

Chu, F. & Trotter, S. *The mental health complex. Part I: Community mental health centers.* Washington, D.C.: Center for Study of Responsive Law, 1972.

Costonis, A. The mental hospital unit system: A critical evaluation and research statement. *J. Health & Human Behavior*, 1966, **7**, 75–83.

Crane, G. Clinical psychopharmacology in its 20th year.

Science, 1973 (July), **181**, 124–128.

Cumming, E. Three issues affecting partnerships among mental health agencies. *Hosp. Comm. Psychiat.*, 1971, **22**, 33–37.

Cumming, J. & Cumming, E. *Ego and milieu.* New York: Atherton Press, 1962.

Demone, H. The limits of rationality in planning. *Comm. Ment. Hlth. J.*, 1965, **1**, 375–381.

Demone, H. Human services at state and local levels and the integration of mental health. In G. Caplan (Ed.), *American handbook of psychiatry* (2nd Ed.), Vol. II. New York: Basic Books, 1974.

Demone, H. & Schulberg, H. Regionalization of health and welfare services. In R. Morris (Ed.), *Encyclopedia of social work* (Sixteenth Issue). New York: National Association of Social Workers, 1971. Pp. 1083–1088.

Deutsch, A. *The shame of the states.* New York: Harcourt, Brace & Co., 1948.

Dill, W. Environment as an influence on managerial autonomy. *Admin. Sci. Quart.*, 1958, **2**, 409–443.

Duhl, F. A personal history of politics and programs in psychiatric training. In G. Abrams & N. Greenfield (Eds.), *The new hospital psychiatry.* New York: Academic Press, 1971. Pp. 7–26.

Dunham, W. Community psychiatry: The newest therapeutic bandwagon. *Arch. Gen. Psychiat.*, 1965, **12**, 303–313.

Duran, F. The unit system— Its effects upon nursing. *J. Psychiat. Nursing*, 1964, **2**, 532–539.

Ellsworth, R., Dickman, H., & Maroney, R. Characteristics of productive and unproductive unit systems in V.A. psychiatric hospitals. *Hosp. Comm. Psychiat.*, 1972, **23**, 261–268.

Ellsworth, R. & Maroney, R. Characteristics of psychiatric programs and their effects on patients' adjustments. *J. Consult. Clin. Psychol.*, 1972, **39**, 436–447.

Emery, F. & Trist, E. Socio-technical systems. In C.W. West-Churchman & M. Verhulst (Eds.), *Management sciences: Models and techniques,* Vol. II. New York: Pergamon Press, 1960.

Emery, F. & Trist, E. The causal texture of organizational environments. *Human Relations*, 1965, **18**, 21–32.

Esquibel, E. & Bower, W. Changeover of a mental hospital unit into a therapeutic community. *Int. J. Group Psychotherapy*, 1965, **15**, 11-16.

Etzioni, A. Two approaches to organizational analysis—A critique and a suggestion. *Admin. Sci. Quart.*, 1960, **5**, 257–278. (a)

Etzioni, A. Interpersonal and structural factors in the study of mental hospitals. *Psychiatry*, 1960, **23**, 13–22. (b)

Etzioni, A. & Lehman, E. Some dangers of "valid" social measurements. *The Annals of the American Academy of Political and Social Science*, 1967, **373**, 1–15.

Evenson, R., Nieuwenhuizen, M., Sletten, I., & Cho, D. A computerized survey of treatments used in Missouri institutions. *Hosp. Comm. Psychiat.*, 1973, **24**, 23–26.

Ewalt, P. *Mental health volunteers.* Springfield, Ill.: Charles C. Thomas, 1967.

Feinsilver, D. & Gunderson, J. Psychotherapy for schizophrenics— Is it indicated? *Schizophrenia Bull.*, Rockville, Md.: NIMH, No. 6, Fall, 1972.

Fischer, A. & Weinstein, M. Mental hospitals, prestige, and the image of enlightenment. *Arch. Gen. Psychiat.*, 1971, **25**, 41–48.

Fisher, M., Mehr, J., & Truckenbrud, P. *Power, greed, and stupidity in the mental health racket.* Philadelphia: Westminster Press, 1973.

Fogelson, F. & Demone, H. Program change through mental health planning. *Comm. Ment. Hlth. J.*, 1969, **5**, 3–13.

Freeman, H. & Simmons, O. *The mental patient comes home.* New York: Wiley & Sons, 1963.

Freidson, E. *Professional dominance: The social structure of medical care.* New York: Atherton Press, 1970.

Garcia, L. The Clarinda Plan: An ecological approach to hospital organization. *Mental Hospitals*, 1960, **11**, 30–31.

Geyerhahn, G. & Mesnick, J. Responses of registered nurses toward community mental health concepts as depicted in the "Community Mental Health Ideology Scale." Unpublished master's thesis. Boston University School of Nursing, 1971.

Gilbert, D. & Levinson, D. "Custodialism" and "humanism" in staff ideology. In M. Greenblatt, D. Levinson, & R. Williams (Eds.), *The patient and the mental hospital.* Glencoe, Ill.: The Free Press, 1957. Pp. 20–36.

Glass, A. The future of large public mental hospitals. *Hosp. Comm. Psychiat.*, 1965, **16**, 9–22.

Glasscote, R. & Kanno, C. *The plans for planning: A comparative analysis of the state mental health planning proposals.* Washington, D.C.: Joint Information Service, 1963.

Glasscote, R., Kraft, A., Glassman, D., & Jepson, W. *Partial hospitalization for the mentally ill.* Washington, D.C.: Joint Information Service, 1969.

Goffman, E. *Asylums: Essays on the social situation of mental patients and other inmates.* Garden City, New York: Doubleday Anchor, 1961.

Goldberg, L., Baker, F., & Rubenstein, A. Local-cosmopolitan: Unidimensional or multidimensional? *Amer. J. Soc.*, 1965, **70**, 704–710.

Goldstein, R., Racy, J., Dressler, D., Ciottone, R., & Willis, J. What benefits patients? *Psychiat. Quart.*,

1972, **46**, 49–80.

Gorman, M. *Every other bed.* Cleveland: World Publishing Co., 1956.

Gottesfeld, H., Lieberman, F., Roen, S., & Gordon, S. Strategies in innovative human service programs. In H. Schulberg, F. Baker, & S. Roen (Eds.), *Developments in human services,* Vol. I. New York: Behavioral Publications, 1973.

Greenblatt, M. University-hospital collaboration in psychiatric education. *Hosp. Comm. Psychiat.*, 1965, **16,** 167–169.

Greenblatt, M. A new image to gladden our hearts. *Amer. J. Psychiat.*, 1966, **123**, 199–200.

Greenblatt, M. The public psychiatric hospital: Room for optimism. *Amer. J. Psychiat.*, 1971, **127**, 1397–1398.

Greenblatt, M. The evolution of state mental hospital models of treatment. In A. Leighton, R. Wilson, & B. Kaplan (Eds.), *Further explorations in social psychiatry*. New York: Basic Books, 1972.

Greenblatt, M., Levinson, D., & Williams, R. (Eds.) *The patient and the mental hospital.* Glencoe, Ill.: The Free Press, 1957.

Greenblatt, M. & Schulberg, H. The mental hospital and its links to community systems. *Canadian Psychiatric Assoc. J.*, 1970, **15**, 615–623.

Greenblatt, M., Sharaf, M., & Stone, E. *Dynamics of institutional change.* Pittsburgh, Pa.: University of Pittsburgh Press, 1971.

Greenblatt, M., York, R., & Brown, E. *From custodial to therapeutic patient care in mental hospitals.* New York: Russell Sage, 1955.

Grinspoon, L., Ewalt, J., & Shader, R. Psychotherapy and pharmacotherapy in chronic schizophrenia. *Amer. J. Psychiat.*, 1968, **124**, 1645–1652.

Grob, G. Samuel B. Woodward and the practice of psychiatry in early nineteenth-century America. *Bull.*

History Medicine, 1962, **36**, 420–443.
Grob, G. *The state and the mentally ill: A history of Worcester State Hospital in Massachusetts, 1830–1920*. Chapel Hill: University of N. Carolina Press, 1966.
Gross, B. *The managing of organizations*. Glencoe, Ill.: Free Press, 1964.
Gross, B. The state of the nation: Social systems accounting. In R. Bauer (Ed.), *Social indicators*. Cambridge, Mass.: MIT Press, 1966.
Gross, H. The Community Mental Health Ideology Scale: Validation. Butler Hospital, Providence, R.I., 1972, mimeographed paper.
Gross, R. A conceptual outline for day treatment center practice. *Comp. Psychiatry*, 1971, **12**, 437–449.
Grunebaum, H. (Ed.) *The practice of community mental health*. Boston: Little, Brown, & Co., 1970.
Haire, M. *Modern organization theory*. New York: Wiley & Sons, 1959.
Hall, A. & Fagen, R. Definition of system. *General Systems Yearbook*, 1956, **1**, 18–28.
Hansell, N. Casualty management method: An aspect of mental health technology in transition. *Arch. Gen. Psychiat.*, 1968, **19**, 281–289.
Hansell, N., Wodarczyk, M., & Visotsky, H. The mental health expediter. *Arch. Gen. Psychiat.*, 1968, **18**, 392–399.
Hefferin, E. & Wilner, D. Opinions about geriatric patients in public mental hospitals. *HSMHA Health Reports*, 1971, **86**, 457–472.
Hersch, C. Social history, mental health, and community control. *Amer. Psychologist*, 1972, **27**, 749–754.
Hirschowitz, R. Dilemmas of leadership in community mental health. *Psychiat. Quart.*, 1971, **45**, 102–116.
Hirschowitz, R. Grand rounds circus. *Social Policy*, 1973, **10**, 50–55(a).

Hirschowitz, R. A model for effective staff deployment in the revitalized mental hospital. *Psychiat. Quart.*, 1973, **47**, 56–70(b).

Hoch, P. Mental hospitals—today and tomorrow. Paper presented at Brockton, Massachusetts V.A. Hospital. April 1, 1964.

Hogarty, G., Goldberg, S., & the Collaborative Study Group. Drug and sociotherapy in the aftercare of schizophrenic patients. *Arch. Gen. Psychiat.*, 1973, **28**, 54–64.

Holder, H. & Stratas, N. A systems approach to alcoholism programming. *Amer. J. Psychiat.*, 1972, **129**, 32–37.

Hollingshead, A. & Redlich, F. *Social class and mental illness.* New York: John Wiley, 1958.

Homans, G. *The human group.* New York: Harcourt, Brace, 1950.

Howard, L. & Baker, F. Ideology and role function of the nurse in community mental health. *Nursing Research*, 1971, **20**, 450–454.

Howe, L. The concept of the community: Some implications for the development of community psychiatry. In L. Bellak (Ed.), *Handbook of community psychiatry and community mental health.* New York: Grune & Stratton, 1964. Pp. 16–46.

Huber, H. Defining the role of the psychiatric nurse. *J. Ft. Logan Mental Health Center,* 1963, **1**, 87–101.

Ishiyama, T. & Grover, W. The phenomenon of resistance to change in a large psychiatric institution. *Psychiat. Quart. Supp.*, 1960, **34**, 1–11.

Jackson, G. & Smith, F. A proposal for mental hospital reorganization: The Kansas Plan. *Mental Hospitals*, 1961, **12**, 5–8.

Jacobs, L. & Kotin, J. Fantasies of psychiatric research. *Amer. J. Psychiat.*, 1972, **128**, 1074–1080.

Jacobson, A. A critical look at the community psychiatric

clinic. *Amer. J. Psychiat.*, 1967 (Oct. supp.), **124**, 14–20.

Jacobson, S., Roman, M., & Kaplan, S. Training nonprofessional workers. In H. Grunebaum (Ed.), *The practice of community mental health.* Boston: Little, Brown, & Co., 1970. Pp. 625–643.

Jepson, W. Metropolitan mental health center development. In H. Grunebaum (Ed.), *The practice of community mental health.* Boston: Little, Brown, & Co., 1970. Pp. 439–467.

Joint Commission on Mental Illness and Health. *Action for mental health.* New York: Basic Books, 1961.

Jones, M. *The therapeutic community.* New York: Basic Books, 1953.

Kantor, D. & Gelineau, V. Making chronic schizophrenics. *Ment. Hyg.*, 1969, **53**, 54–66.

Kaplan, H. Institutions and community mental health: The paradox in Wyatt v. Stickney. *Comm. Ment. Hlth. J.*, 1973, **9**, 34–37.

Kaplan, S., Boyajian, L., & Meltzer, B. The role of the nonprofessional worker. In H. Grunebaum (Ed.), *The practice of community mental health.* Boston: Little, Brown, & Co., 1970. Pp. 591–624.

Katz, D. The motivational basis of organizational behavior. *Behavioral Science*, 1964, **9**, 131–146.

Katz, D. & Kahn, R. *The social psychology of organizations.* New York: Wiley & Sons, 1966.

Kazdin, A. & Bootzin, R. The token economy: An evaluative review. *J. Applied Behavioral Analysis*, 1972, **5**, 343–372.

Kelly, J. Ecological constraints on mental health services. *Amer. Psychologist*, 1966, **21**, 535–539.

Kempler, H. Positive organizational change in a mental health setting: A case study. Presented at Annual Meeting of the American Orthopsychiatric Association, Washington, D.C., 1971.

Kiger, R. Adopting the unit plan: I. Processes. *Hosp.*

Comm. Psychiat., 1966, **17**, 207–212.

Killian, L. Social movements. In R. Faris (Ed.), *Handbook of modern sociology.* Chicago, Ill.: Rand McNally, 1964. Pp. 426–455.

Klein, D. *Community dynamics and mental health.* New York: Wiley & Sons, 1968.

Kotin, J. & Schur, M. Attitudes of discharged mental patients toward their hospital experiences. *J. Nerv. Ment. Dis.*, 1969, **149**, 408–414.

Kotin, J. & Sharaf, M. Intrastaff controversy at a state mental hospital: An analysis of ideological issues. *Psychiatry*, 1967, **30**, 16–19. (a)

Kotin, J. & Sharaf, M. Management succession and administrative style. *Psychiatry*, 1967, **30**, 237–248. (b)

Kraft, A. Fort Logan Mental Health Center—A progress report. *Mental Hospitals*, 1963, **14**, 534–535.

Kraft, A., Binner, P., & Dickey, B. The community mental health program and the longer-stay patient. *Arch. Gen. Psychiat.*, 1967, **16**, 64–70.

Kris, A. & Schiff, L. An adolescent consultation service in a state mental hospital: Maintaining treatment motivation. *Seminars in Psychiatry*, 1969, **1**, 15–23.

Kris, A., Schiff, L., & McLaughlin, R. Susceptibility to chronic hospitalization relative to age at first admission. *Arch. Gen. Psychiat.*, 1971, **24**, 346–352.

Lamb, H. & Goertzel, V. Discharged mental patients—Are they really in the community? *Arch. Gen. Psychiat.*, 1971, **24**, 29–34.

Lamb, H. & Goertzel, V. The demise of the state hospital—A premature obituary? *Arch. Gen. Psychiat.*, 1972, **26**, 489–495.

Langston, R. Community mental health centers and community mental health ideology. *Comm. Ment. Hlth. J.*, 1970, **6**, 387–392.

Lanyon, R. Mental health technology. *Amer. Psychologist*,

1971, **26**, 1071–1076.

Lawrence, P. & Lorsch, J. Differentiation and integration in complex organizations. *Admin. Sci. Quart.*, 1967, **12**, 1–47.

Lehmann, S. Community and psychology and community psychology. *Amer. Psychologist*, 1971, **26**, 554–560.

Leopold, R. The West Philadelphia mental health consortium: Administrative planning in a multihospital catchment area. *Amer. J. Psychiat.*, 1967 (Oct. supp.), **124**, 69–76.

Levenson, A. Staffing. In H. Grunebaum (Ed.), *The practice of community mental health.* Boston: Little, Brown, & Co., 1970. Pp. 551–570.

Levine, M. & Levine, A. *A social history of helping services: Clinic, court, school and community.* New York: Appleton-Century-Crofts, 1970.

Levinson, D. Role, personality, and social structure in the organizational setting. *J. Abnorm. Soc. Psychol.*, 1959, **58**, 170–180.

Levinson, D. Idea systems in the individual and society. In G. Zollschan & W. Hirsch (Eds.), *Explorations in social change.* Boston: Houghton Mifflin, 1964. Pp. 297–318.

Levy, L. The state mental hospital in transition: A review of principles. *Comm. Ment. Hlth. J.*, 1965, **1**, 353–356.

Linn, L. Measuring the effectiveness of mental hospitals. *Hosp. Comm. Psychiat.*, 1970, **21**, 381–386.

Loeb, M. Community psychiatry: What it is and what it is not. In L. Roberts, S. Halleck, & M. Loeb (Eds.), *Community psychiatry.* Madison, Wisconsin: University of Wisconsin Press, 1966. Pp. 223–236.

London, P. The end of ideology in behavior modification. *Amer. Psychologist*, 1972, **27**, 913–920.

Lorei, T. Staff ratings of the relative importance of the consequences of release from or retention in a psychiatric hospital. *J. Consult. Clin. Psychol.*, 1970, **34**, 48–55.

Lorei, T. & Gurel, L. Demographic characteristics as predictors of posthospital employment and readmission. *J. Consult. Clin. Psychol., 1973*, **40**, 426–430.

March, M. The neighborhood center concept. *Public Welfare,* 1968, **26**, 97–111.

Martin, H. Inside the insane asylum. *Saturday Evening Post*, April 6, 1968, 32–47.

Massachusetts Mental Health Planning Project. *Mental health for Massachusetts.* Boston, Mass.: Massachusetts Department of Mental Health, 1965.

May, P. *Treatment of schizophrenia.* New York: Science House, 1968.

May, P., Yale, C., & Dixon, W. Assessment of psychiatric outcome— I. Cross section analysis. *J. Psychiat. Res.*, 1972, **9**, 271–284.

Mendel, W. On the abolition of the psychiatric hospital. In L. Roberts, N. Greenfield, & M. Miller (Eds.), *Comprehensive mental health: The challenge of evaluation.* Madison, Wis.: University of Wisconsin Press, 1968. Pp. 237–247.

Mental Health Association of Southeastern Pennsylvania. *The unit plan conference transcript,* Philadelphia, Pa., February 25, 1963.

Merton, R. *Social theory and social structure.* Glencoe, Ill.: The Free Press, 1957.

Milbank Memorial Fund. Decentralization of mental hospitals. *Milbank Memorial Fund Quart.*, 1964, **42**, 115–177.

Mill, C. Interprofessional awareness of roles. *J. Clin. Psych.*, 1960, **16**, 411–413.

Miller, J. Living systems: Basic concepts. *Behavioral Science*, 1965, **10**, 193–237. (a)

Miller, J. Living systems: Structure and process. *Behavioral Science*, 1965, **10**, 337–379. (b)

Mirelowitz, S. Alienation and bureaucratization of mental health organizations. *Ment. Hyg.*, 1972, **56**, 6–12.

Morton, W., Lantz, A., & Halpern, J. Readmissions: Methodology and meaning. *J. Ft. Logan Mental Health Center*, 1970, **6**, 1–22.

Mosher, L. & Gunderson, J. Special report: Schizophrenia, 1972. *Schizophrenia Bull.*, Rockville, Md.: NIMH, No. 7, Winter, 1973.

Myerson, D. Can institutionalization be prevented? *Mass. J. Ment. Hlth.*, 1972, **2**, 17–26.

National Institute of Mental Health. Patients in state and county mental hospitals, 1967. Washington, D.C.: U.S. Govt. Printing Office, PHS Publication No. 1921, 1969.

Oberleder, M. A state hospital closes its doors to the elderly. *Gerontologist*, 1973, **13**, 45–49.

O'Neill, F. The mental hospital: Cornerstone for community psychiatric services. *Amer. J. Psychiat.*, 1960, **116**, 810–813.

Overall, J. & Henry, B. Decisions about drug therapy: III. Selection of treatment for psychiatric inpatients. *Arch. Gen. Psychiat.*, 1973, **28**, 81–89.

Ozarin, L. & Feldman, S. Implications for health service delivery: The Community Mental Health Centers Amendments of 1970. *Amer. J. Pub. Hlth.*, 1971, **61**, 1780–1784.

Ozarin, L. & Levenson, A. The future of the public mental hospital. *Amer. J. Psychiat.*, 1969, **125**, 1647–1652.

Panzetta, A. *Community mental health: Myth and reality.* Philadelphia: Lea & Febiger, 1971.(a)

Panzetta, A. The concept of community. *Arch. Gen. Psy-*

chiat., 1971, **25**, 291–297.(b)

Pasamanick, B., Scarpitti, F., & Dinitz, S. *Schizophrenics in the community.* New York: Appleton-Century-Crofts, 1967.

Pattison, E. & Elpers, J. A developmental view of mental health manpower trends. *Hosp. Comm. Psychiat.*, 1972, **23**, 325–328.

Peck, H., Roman, M., & Kaplan, S. Community action programs and the comprehensive mental health center. In M. Greenblatt, P. Emery, & B. Glueck (Eds.), *Poverty and mental health.* Washington, D.C.: American Psychiatric Association, 1967. Pp. 103–121.

Penn, N., Baker, F., & Schulberg, H. Community mental health ideology and personality preferences. Unpublished paper, 1973. (a)

Penn, N., Baker, F., & Schulberg, H. Survey of community mental health attitudes among social work students. Unpublished paper, 1973. (b)

Pepper, M. Reorganization of the mental hospital. *Gerontologist*, 1964, **4**, 53–57.

Perrow, C. Hospitals: Technology, structure, and goals. In J. March (Ed.), *Handbook of organizations.* Chicago, Ill.: Rand McNally, 1965. Pp. 910–971.

Pokorny, A. & Bentinck, C. A study of relatives' views of state mental hospital patients. *Social Casework*, 1969, **50**, 519–526.

Polak, P. The irrelevance of hospital treatment to the patient's social system. *Hosp. Comm. Psychiat.*, 1971, **22**, 255–256.

Polak, P. & Jones, M. The psychiatric nonhospital: A model for change. *Comm. Ment. Hlth. J.*, 1973, **9**, 123–132.

Psychiatric News. California to phase out mental hospitals by 1982. *Psychiatric News,* Vol. **8**, No. 8, April 18, 1973.(a)

Psychiatric News. Alabama struggles to meet court-imposed mental hospital standards, *Psychiatric News,* Vol. **8**, No. 10, May 16, 1973.(b)

Rabkin, J. Opinions about mental illness: A review of the literature. *Psychol. Bull.*, 1972, **77**, 153–171.

Rapaport, M. Mental hospital research at a state hospital: An attempt at a balanced program. *Ment. Hyg.*, 1968, **52**, 110–123.

Rice, A. *The enterprise and its environment.* London: Tavistock, 1963.

Rokeach, M. *The open and closed mind.* New York: Basic Books, 1960.

Rosenblum, G. & Ottenstein, D. From child guidance to community mental health: Problems in transition. *Comm. Ment. Hlth. J.*, 1965, **1**, 276–283.

Rowitz, L. & Levy, L. The state mental hospital in transition: An approach to the study of mental hospital decentralization. *Ment. Hyg.*, 1971, **55**, 68–76.

Rushing, W. *The psychiatric professions: Power, conflict, and adaptation in a psychiatric hospital staff.* Chapel Hill: University of North Carolina Press, 1964.

Ryan, W. *Blaming the victim.* New York: Vintage Books, 1972.

Schiff, S. A therapeutic community in an open state hospital: Administrative framework for social psychiatry. *Hosp. Comm. Psychiat.,* 1969, **20**, 259–268.

Schulberg, H. State planning for community mental health programs: Implications for psychologists. *Comm. Ment. Hlth. J.*, 1965, **1**, 37–42.

Schulberg, H. Future steps in implementing mental health plans. *Comm. Ment. Hlth. J.*, 1966, **2**, 157–162. (a)

Schulberg, H. Private practice and community mental health. *Hosp. Comm. Psychiat.*, 1966, **17**, 363–366. (b)

Schulberg, H. Community mental health: Fact or fiction? *Canada's Mental Health*, 1969 (Nov.–Dec.),

Supp. 63.
Schulberg, H. The challenge of human service programs for psychologists. *Amer. Psychologist*, 1972, **27**, 566–573.
Schulberg, H. The mental hospital in the era of human services. *Hosp. Comm. Psychiat.*, 1973, **24**, 467–472.
Schulberg, H. & Baker, F. Varied attitudes to community mental health. *Arch. Gen. Psychiat.*, 1967, **17**, 658–663.
Schulberg, H. & Baker, F. Community mental health: The belief system of the 1960's. *Psychiat. Opinion*, 1969 (April), **6**, 14–26. (a)
Schulberg, H. & Baker, F. Unitization: Decentralizing the mental hospitalopolis. *Int. J. Psychiat.*, 1969, **7**, 213–223. (b)
Schulberg, H. & Baker, F. Interprofessional relations. In H. Grunebaum (Ed.), *The practice of community mental health.* Boston: Little, Brown, & Co., 1970. Pp. 645–662. (a)
Schulberg, H. & Baker, F. The caregiving system in community mental health programs: An application of open-systems theory. *Com. Ment. Hlth. J.*, 1970, **6**, 437–446. (b)
Schulberg, H. & Baker, F. The history and development of Boston State Hospital: 1839 to 1963. *Mass. J. Ment. Hlth.*, 1971, **2**, 20–30.
Schulberg, H., Baker, F., & Roen, S. (Eds.) *Developments in human services*, Vol. I. New York: Behavioral Publications, 1973.
Schulberg, H. & Demone, H. The impact of mental health planning. *Psychiat. Digest*, 1966, **27**, 33–41.
Schulberg, H., Notman, R., & Bookin, E. Treatment services at a mental hospital in transition. *Amer. J. Psychiat.*, 1967, **124**, 506–513.
Schulberg, H., Sheldon, A., & Baker, F. (Eds.) *Program evaluation in the health fields.* New York: Behavioral

Schulberg, H. & Wechsler, H. The uses and misuses of data in assessing mental health needs. *Comm. Ment. Hlth. J.*, 1967, **3**, 389–395.
Publications, 1969.

Schulberg, H. & Wojcik, S. A reanalysis of treatment at a changing mental hospital. *Hosp. Comm. Psychiat.*, 1971, **22**, 19–23.

Sharaf, M., Kaplan, R., & Cole, J. Developing a community mental health center in a large state hospital: Some problematic issues. *Mass. J. Ment. Hlth.*, 1971, **1**, 19–27.

Sharaf, M. & Levinson, D. Patterns of ideology and role differentiation among psychiatric residents. In M. Greenblatt, D. Levinson, & R. Williams (Eds.), *The patient and the mental hospital.* Glencoe, Ill.: The Free Press, 1957. Pp. 263–285.

Shaw, R. & Eagle, C. Programmed failure: The Lincoln Hospital story. *Comm. Ment. Hlth. J.*, 1971, **7**, 255–263.

Sheffel, I. Non-medical administrators—colleagues, not rivals. *Hosp. Comm. Psychiat.*, 1967, **18**, 129–134.

Smith, H. Mental hospital organization: Challenge and response. *Mental Hospitals*, 1964, **15**, 67–71.

Smith, T., Bower, W., & Wignall, C. Influence of policy and drugs on Colorado State Hospital population. *Arch. Gen. Psychiat.*, 1965, **12**, 352–362.

Snow, H. Aspects of decentralization of a state hospital. *Psychiat. Quart.*, 1965, **39**, 607–620.

Solomon, H. The American Psychiatric Association in relation to American psychiatry. *Amer. J. Psychiat.*, 1958, **115**, 1–9.

Spadoni, A. & Smith, J. Milieu therapy in schizophrenia. *Arch. Gen. Psychiat.*, 1969, **20**, 547–551.

Stanton, A. & Schwartz, M. *The mental hospital.* New York: Basic Books, 1954.

Stewart, A., LaFave, H., Grunberg, F., & Herjanic, M. Problems in phasing out a large public psychiatric

hospital. *Amer. J. Psychiat.*, 1968, **125**, 82–88.
Stotsky, B. The psychiatric patient in the nursing home: A retrospective study. *J. Amer. Geriatrics Soc.*, 1966, **14**, 735–747. (a)
Stotsky, B. Nursing homes: A review. *Amer. J. Psychiat.*, 1966, **123**, 249–258. (b)
Stotsky, B. Are state mental hospitals dumping aged patients on nursing homes? *Comm. Ment. Hlth. J.*, 1968, **4**, 53–61.
Stotsky, B. Social and clinical issues in geriatric psychiatry. *Amer. J. Psychiat.*, 1972, **129**, 117–126.
Stotsky, B. & Margolin, R. Positive and negative factors in the therapeutic community. *Dis. Nerv. Sys.*, 1967, **28**, 19–25.
Stratton, D. & Barton, W. The geriatric patient in the public mental hospital. *Geriatrics*, 1964, **19**, 55–60.
Strauss, A., Schatzman, L., Bucher, R., Ehrlich, D., & Sabshin, M. *Psychiatric ideologies and institutions.* New York: The Free Press of Glencoe, 1964.
Stubblebine, J. & Decker, J. Are urban mental health centers worth it? *Amer. J. Psychiat.*, 1971, **127**, 908–912.
Szasz, T. Hospital-patient relationships in medicine and psychiatry. *Ment. Hyg.*, 1961, **45**, 171–179.
Terreberry, S. The evolution of organizational environments. *Admin. Sci. Quart.*, 1968, **12**, 590–613.
Thompson, J. & McEwan, W. Organizational goals and environment: Goal-setting as an interaction process. *Amer. Soc. Review*, 1958, **23**, 23–31.
Time Magazine. Journey through two Americas: Dorchester-Mattapan, Massachusetts. April 6, 1970, 30.
Trist, E. & Bamforth, K. Some social and psychological consequences of the long-wall method of goal-setting. *Human Relations,* 1961, **4**, 3–38.
Trist, E., Higgin, G., Murray, H., & Pollack, A. *Organiza-*

tional choice. London: Tavistock, 1963.

Ullmann, L. *Institution and outcome: A comparative study of psychiatric hospitals.* New York: Pergamon Press, 1967.

U.S. Department of Health, Education, and Welfare, Public Health Service. Planning of facilities for mental health services. Public Health Service Publication No. 808, Washington, D.C., U.S. Govt. Printing Office, January, 1961.

U.S. Department of Health, Education, and Welfare, Public Health Service, National Institute of Mental Health. Digest state mental health planning grant proposals 1963. Bethesda, Md., 1963. (a)

U.S. Department of Health, Education, and Welfare, Public Health Service, National Institute of Mental Health. Guidelines for the federal grant-in-aid program to support mental health planning. Bethesda, Md., January 22, 1963. (b)

U.S. Department of Health, Education, and Welfare. Regulations: Community Mental Health Centers Act 1963. *Federal Register*, May 6, 1964.

Vacchiano, R., Strauss, P., & Schiffman, D. Personality correlates of dogmatism. *J. Clin. Consult. Psychol.*, 1968, **32**, 83–85.

Vidaver, R. Developments in human services education and manpower. In H. Schulberg, F. Baker, & S. Roen (Eds.), *Developments in human services.* Vol. 1. New York: Behavioral Publications, 1973. Pp. 508–524.

Weiner, L., Becker, A., & Friedman, T. *Home treatment: Spearhead of community psychiatry.* Pittsburgh: University of Pittsburgh Press, 1967.

Wessen, A. Hospital ideology and communication between ward and personnel. In E. Jaco (Ed.), *Patients, physicians, and illness.* Glencoe, Ill.: The Free Press, 1958.

Whittington, H. The ideational basis of a state program for community mental health services. In L. Roberts, S. Halleck, & M. Loeb (Eds.), *Community psychiatry.* Garden City, N.Y.: Anchor Books, 1969. Pp. 119–137.

Wilder, J., Levin, G., & Zwerling, I. A two-year follow-up evaluation of acute psychiatric patients treated in a day hospital. *Amer. J. Psychiat.*, 1966, **122**, 1095–1101.

Wolford, J., Hitchcock, J., Ellison, D., Sonis, A., & Smith, F. The effect on state hospitalization of a community mental health/mental retardation center. *Amer. J. Psychiat.*, 1972, **129**, 202–206.

Yolles, S. The role of the psychologist in comprehensive community mental health centers: The NIMH point of view. *Amer. Psychologist*, 1966, **21**, 37–41.

Yuchtman, E. & Seashore, S. A system resource approach to organizational effectiveness. *Amer. Soc. Review*, 1967, **32**, 891–903.

Zander, A., Cohen, A., & Stotland, E. *Role relations in the mental health professions.* Ann Arbor: University of Michigan Press, 1957.

Zeitlyn, B. The therapeutic community— fact or fantasy? *Brit. J. Psychiat.*, 1967, **113**, 1083–1086.

Zubowicz, G. The Kansas modified unit plan. *Hosp. Comm. Psychiat.*, 1967, **18**, 44–46.

Zusman, J. Mental health service quality control: An idea whose time has come. *Comp. Psychiat.*, 1972, **13**, 497–506.

Zwerling, I. & Wilder, J. An evaluation of the applicability of the day hospital in treatment of acutely disturbed patients. *Israel Annals Psychiat.*, 1964, **2**, 162–185.

Author Index

Subject Index